Bircher-Benner Manuals

Manual for prevention of dementia and Alzheimer's disease

Dietary instructions
for their prevention and healing,
with recipes,
detailed advice
and a treatment plan
from a medical centre
dedicated to state-of-the-art healing

Dr. med. Andres Bircher
and colleagues of the
Bircher-Benner Medical Centre,
Lilli Bircher, Pascal Bircher
Anne-Cécile Bircher

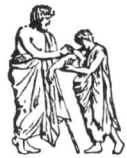

EDITION BIRCHER-BENNER
CH-8784 BRAUNWALD

Bircher-Benner Manuals

1. Manual for patients with multiple sclerosis, Parkinson's disease and other neuro-degenerative diseases
2. Manual for patients with liver and gallbladder conditions
3. Manual for families and children
4. Manual of fresh juices, raw vegetables and fruit dishes
5. Manual for improvement of the immune-system and against susceptibility to infection
6. Manual for mountaineers and athletes
7. Manual for diabetics
8. Manual for support and preventive therapy for lung diseases
9. Enjoying recipes without table salt
10. Manual for patients with rheumatism and arthritis
11. Manual for men with prostate conditions
12. Manual for patients with kidney and bladder conditions
13. Manual for venous diseases
14. Manual for patients with gastro-intestinal conditions
15. Manual for nutrition during pregnancy and lactation
16. Manual for gynaecological problems and menopause
17. Manual for the prevention of cancer and accompanying therapies
18. Manual for headache and migraine
19. Manual for patients with hypertension, cardiovascular disease and arterio-sclerosis
20. Manual for overcoming anxiety and depression
21. Manual for patients with skin diseases or sensitive skin
22. Manual for persons suffering from stress
23. Manual for persons suffering from allergies
24. Manual for prevention of dementia and Alzheimer's disease
25. Manual for internal treatment of eye problems
26. Manual for treatment of weight problems, overweight, and anorexia

These manuals are the result of global research, the development of the art and science of medicine over more than a century, and the experience of the renowned Bircher-Benner Clinic. The reader will benefit from the helpful support of the well-informed physician every step of the way.

1st edition, 2018

All rights reserved, including the right of reproduction in excerpts, photomechanical reproduction and translation
info@bircher-benner.com   www.bircher-benner.com

Book orders: edition@bircher-benner.com
© Copyright by Edition Bircher-Benner, CH 8784 Braunwald
® The trademarks Bircher and Bircher-Benner are protected worldwide
Printed in Germany

The suggestions in this book have been carefully reviewed by the authors and the publisher. However, we cannot assume any guarantee. The authors and the publisher hereby disclaim all liability for personal injury, property damage and any type of financial loss.

Cover design: Kösel Media GmbH, Krugzell. Germany
Overall production: Kösel GmbH, Krugzell. Germany

Table of Contents

Preface 7

Introduction 9

The structure of the central nervous system 10
    The cerebrum 10
    The cerebellum 11
    The pons 11
    The basal ganglia 11
    The thalamic nucleus 11
    The substantia nigra 12
    The limbic system 12
    The motor pathways 12
    The sensitive tracks 13
    The hormone-producing glands of the brain 13
    The posterior pituitary (neurohypophysis) 14
    The epiphysis and melatonin 14
    The nerve cell (neuron) 14
    The potential for action 15
    The synapses 15
    Inhibiting messenger substances 16
    The importance of the glial cells in the brain 16
    The spaces of the brain and the fluid in the brain and spinal cord 17
    The blood-brain barrier 17

The myelin marrow sheaths – a sensitive substance 22

Demyelinating diseases 23

Remyelination 24

Diseases from storage of degenerative proteins	25
The TAU proteins	25
Amyloidosis	25
The effect of nutrition on the central nervous system	27
Two kinds of food energy	27
The basic regulation system of the soft connective tissue in the central nervous system	29
Oxidative stress at the centre of the causes of neurodegenerative diseases	31
The influence of environmental stress from pollutants as the cause of neurogenerative diseases	33
The neurotoxic effect of mercury	33
Organic tin compounds and neurodegeneration	34
Chlorine and neurodegenerative diseases	35
The neurotoxic effect of volatile organic hydrocarbons	36
Pesticides and neurodegenerative diseases	36
Wood-protection agents and neurodegenerative diseases	37
Neurotoxic medicines and neurodegeneration	37
Legal and prohibited drugs and neurodegenerative diseases	39
Cannabis	39
Amphetamines	39
LSD (lysergic acid diethylamide)	39
Heroin, morphine, other opiates	40
Cocaine	40
Nicotine	40
Alcohol	41
Caffeine	41
Regarding the phenomenon of primary and secondary effects and the danger of polypragmasia from medication	42
The combined effect of harmful neurotoxic substances	42
Vitamins, trace elements and neurodegenerative disease	44
The diversity of causes of neurodegenerative diseases	46

The various types of neurodegenerative diseases	47
Systematic overview of neurodegenerative diseases	47
Dementia	49
Diagnosis of dementia	49
Forms of dementia	49
Dementia becomes more and more frequent	50
Officially accepted risk factors of dementia	50
The symptoms of dementia	51
Diagnosis of dementia	52
Notes on care and nursing for persons suffering from dementia	52
Alzheimer's disease	57
Causes of Alzheimer's disease	57
What happens in the brain at Alzheimer's disease	59
The symptoms of Alzheimer's disease	60
The stages of the disease	60
Diagnosis of Alzheimer's disease	60
Not every memory loss in old age is equivalent to Alzheimer's disease	61
The early and medium stages of Alzheimer's disease	61
The later stage of Alzheimer's disease	61
Change of character by Alzheimer's disease	61
Physical deterioration of patients with Alzheimer's disease	62
Life expectancy at Alzheimer's disease	62
Prophylaxis and treatment of Alzheimer's disease	62
The officially recognised risk factors of Alzheimer's disease	64
Order therapy for Alzheimer's disease	64
Dietary treatment of neurodegenerative diseases	65
Lab control recommendations for the attending physician during the diet	68
Practical application of the raw food therapy	72
Menus	72
Daily Menu	74
The Recipes	76

Juices	76
Bircher muesli	77
Fruit and fresh grain dishes	78
Chilled soups	79
Milk types	79
Raw vegetables and salads	80
Salad dressings	81
Suggestions for dressings to go with the salads and raw vegetables	83
Cooked food	84
Recipes for cooked food	85
Vegetables	88
Salads of cooked vegetables	92
Potato dishes	93
Cereal dishes	94
Sauces	97
Sandwiches	99
Desserts	100
Recipes	104
Notes	107
Index	115

Preface

Dementia brings unspeakable suffering to people. Challenged by life, after we have achieved a lot, lived through a lot and were happily looking forward to a calm, well-deserved retirement, it mercilessly takes hold of us and robs us of our wits. We no longer understand the world around us, not our relatives and not even ourselves. Seized by fear and illusions, we lose all trust in ourselves, trust in those who once respected us, who gave us safety and a home. Our distress grows greater and greater until we can no longer even take care of ourselves or do our everyday work, surrounded by people whose names we cannot remember, whom we barely recognise, even if they are our own children.

When German psychiatrist and neuropathologist Alois Alzheimer first described 'a strange case of dementia, a strange disease of the cerebral cortex' in 1906, he hardly received any attention at all. Today the disease is widespread and feared.

There is no consensus on the cause. However, it is impossible to miss that there is a continuous increase of Alzheimer's disease, of vascular dementia and of Parkinson's disease in all Western countries.

In all frequent forms of dementia, Alzheimer's disease, vascular dementia, Lewy body dementia, which occurs in the scope of Parkinson's disease, and in the rarer multiple system atrophy (MSA), genetics barely plays a role. Discounting Parkinson's disease and multiple system atrophy, about two-thirds of those suffering from dementia suffer from Alzheimer's and one-third from vascular dementia.

Neurodegenerative diseases usually progress slowly, with degenerative inflammatory processes in various parts of the nervous system. In the last thirty years, numerous papers have identified an increasing number of partial causes of Alzheimer's disease. Vascular dementia results from arteriosclerosis, occlusion of vessels, embolisms and bleeding in the brain. Alzheimer's disease essentially follows the same risk factors as arteriosclerosis. They are the effects of the widespread un-natural lifestyle and nutrition, lack of movement and speed, and most of all unnatural, industrially synthesised foods with an over-abundance of animal products such as meat, eggs and fatty cheese, a lack of polyunsaturated vegetable oils and vitamins A, B, C, D, E and folic acid, and a lack of antioxidant and anti-inflammatory secondary plant substances (Phytochemicals) and fresh, raw, living plant-based food with a high oxidative stress. For Alzheimer's disease and Lewy body dementia of those suffering from Par-kinson's disease, the stress from environmental toxins, such as heavy metals, pesticides, irritants, drugs and medicines that they have taken in dangerous amounts, today has a high causative relevance.

The focus of scientific medical thinking is on the autoimmune processes, i.e. the destructive attacks of the immune system on the structures of the body's nervous system, the nerve cells and the sensitive myelin-containing nerve sheaths. This explains why all therapeutic efforts to combat, for example, multiple sclerosis are focused on medication designed to suppress pathogenic autoimmune inflammation. In Alzheimer's disease, oxidative processes are at the centre, rendering certain proteins insoluble by phosphorylation so that they will deposit in the intercellular tissue and the nerve cells and destroy them. Billions are spent on unsuccessful research for medicines to prevent degenerative phosphorylation. However, very little is spent to research the actual causes of Alzheimer's disease and on treating them. In spite of the immense financial efforts made for medical-pharmacological research, the disease continues to spread, and it is becoming more and more common.

However, medical science has recently started taking the great spatial epidemiological differences in the frequency of Alzheimer's and Parkinson's disease seriously and to understand them. They have recognised that these diseases cannot be explained by genetics, but by differences in nutrition and lifestyle and the environmental conditions. All of these data and many scientific studies strongly suggest that the poor nutrition common in Western industrialised countries is the cause. The causes, prevention and treatment of multiple sclerosis, amyotrophic lateral sclerosis, Guillain-Barré syndrome and Parkinson's disease are described in Bircher-Benner manual no. 1.

This book is based on all the modern scientific insights that are relevant for the understanding, prevention and effective causative treatment of dementia, in addition to more than a century of medical experience. Our greatest teachers are the many patients who have been successfully treated at the famous Bircher-Benner Clinic in Zürich and at our medical centre over the years with our vital vegan fresh food diet, new life order and the careful elimination of toxin stress, foci of diseases and interference fields. This book provides the patient and his family with practical instructions for preventing dementia, or for positively influencing their courses once they have already developed. For the treating physician, this book is a great help for the instruction and guidance of his patients.

Introduction

To understand the causes of Alzheimer's dementia and other neurodegenerative diseases, to the extent to which that they are known today, it is important to have some basic knowledge regarding the construction and function of the central nervous system. In fact, multiple sclerosis may attack and damage the central nervous system anywhere. Therefore its forms are very diverse. Parkinson's disease by contrast has a much more consistent course, since the Nucleus niger, a pigmented core of the basal ganglia of the brain, is always at the centre of destruction by α synuclein here, degenerating before dementia becomes evident. Amyotrophic lateral sclerosis also follows a typical course, since it almost exclusively affects the motoric nerve pathways that are responsible for muscle strength and action and therefore causes increasing paralysis. Vascular dementia shows a different appearance and is usually associated with paralysis corresponding to the location of the vascular occlusions or bleeding. Alzheimer's dementia generally occurs in the entire brain, with the hippocampus and limbic system being particularly affected at first.

These are particularly important for memory. Multiple system atrophy (MSA) takes a particularly quick and tragic course. The dege-nerative progresses also affect the entire brain.

The explanations concerning some of the anatomical and functional situations in the central nervous system help to reveal the causes of these diseases and enable every sensible patient and his family to actively contribute in preventing and healing multiple sclerosis, to the extent this is still possible. This is a very rewarding undertaking.

The structure of the central nervous system

Estimates suggest that the human brain is made up of nearly 100 billion nerve cells (neurons). The number of glial cells (i.e. the cells that protect and feed the nerve cells that keep the living conditions of the neurons constant and that are part of the immune system of the brain) is similarly large.

The cerebrum

The largest number of nerve cells is located in the cerebrum, embedded in the connective-tissue-like supporting framework of the glial cells, in many windings (gyri) and furrows (sulci). The cerebrum is divided into the frontal lobes, the temporal lobes and the occipital cortex. There is a deep furrow on either side (sulcus centralis). The frontal parts of the cerebrum in front of this furrow mostly serve action-related purposes (executive cortex), while those behind it are assigned to sensitivity, perception and sensation. The foremost part of the frontal lobe (pre-frontal cortex) contains the key structure for a circuit that controls decisions and considers whether a decision should be taken in view of potential benefits and dis-advantages. The other convolutions of the brain in the frontal lobe (lobus frontalis) are important for personality development, for clearly focused thinking and for problem-solving skills[1].

The convolution directly in front of the central furrow contains the nerve cells for all movements, like an inverted 'little man' or homunculus (homunculus, motor cortex), with a particularly large number of neurons assigned to the tongue, the hands and feet. If these were stimulated, the body would respond by moving the respective limb on the other side of the body. If the nerve cells in the temporal lobe were stimulated, the body would respond with complex spontaneous movements. Behind the central furrow, there are nerve cells that receive sensations from all body regions (sensory cortex). The left temporal lobe contains cell formations that permit speech (Broca's area and Wernicke's area). The frontal lobes are important for focused, targeted thinking and decision-making, and for guiding and controlling emotions and urges. The occipital cortex contains the centre of visual perception through the eyes (visual cortex).

There are two long protrusions at the front beneath the frontal lobe. This is the olfactory bulb, which is directly connected to olfactory cells.

The nerve cells of the cerebral cortex are grey (grey matter). The nerve fibres (neurites) leading away from them consists of white matter. This matter is white because its nerve fibres are surrounded by lipid-containing (fatty) marrow sheathes that appear white. They protect the nerve fibres (axons) and provide much faster conduction of nerve impulses. The two halves of the cerebrum are linked closely to each other by white nerve fibres. This connection is called the corpus callosum. Below this on both sides is a very primal part of the brain, which is re-miniscent of a sea horse in shape (hippocampus). The hippocampus is where information from different sensation-processing systems (sensory systems) is brought together, processed and returned to the cerebral cortex. The hippocampus is very important for strengthening the memory (i.e. for transferring contents from short-term memory to long-term memory), thereby producing the capacity of memory. After severe emotional trauma, such as war or the consequences of sexual abuse, the hippocampus may shrink (atrophy). However, it has been proven that the neurons in the hippocampus are able to regenerate given the right conditions.

The cerebellum

The cerebellum is located on either side below the occipital lobes. Its primary function is to coordinate movement and walking. The cerebellum and the "bridge" (pons) are collectively called the hindbrain (metencephalon). The pons is a bulge of nerve fibres between the midbrain (mesencephalon) and the afterbrain (myelencephalon). The pons and the myelencephalon form the brain stem, from which the medulla oblongata leads down to the spinal cord.

The pons

The pons is the passage for all pathways that interconnect the 'upstream' and 'downstream' areas of the central nervous system, such as the cerebrum areas to the spinal cord (tractus cerebrospinalis). The pons contains collections of nerve cells (nuclei pontis) that connect the cerebrum to the cerebellum during decussation. The medulla oblongata contains nerve cell collections (nuclei) that control the vital functions, respiration and the heart (respiratory and cardiac centres).

The basal ganglia

Deep inside, between the hemispheres of the cerebrum, are the basal ganglia. They are considered to be part of the cerebrum. Part of them, the 'striped' core (corpus striatum), is divided into the pale core (globus pallidus) and a longitudinal core with a head and a tail (caudate nucleus). The large pathways from the cerebral cortex to the spinal cord run between these. The corpus striatum is a large switchboard that takes in information from the cerebral cortex and controls it by inhibition, like a coachman controlling his horse, and passes it on to the black core (nucleus niger), which in turn controls movements and coordination by inhibition and passes on its information to the thalamus.

The thalamic nucleus

The thalamic nucleus is the 'gate to the conscious mind'. All information emanating from the cells and the sensory cells of the body, the cerebrum and the basal ganglia, are routed towards it. The thalamus selects the information to be supplied to the conscious mind and therefore forwarded to the cerebrum. The thalamus does not work autonomously, but rather is subject to the strict control of the cerebrum. Therefore we speak of the corticothalamic system in the context of the development of consciousness. The visual and auditory pathways from the eye and the inner ear are also connected via the thalamus, except for the olfactory bulb, which has pathways that go straight to the cerebral cortex. The corticothalamic system regulates the sleeping-waking rhythm and the general activity level of the cerebrum, as well as the vegetative nervous system, and controls general protective reflexes such as breathing, swallowing, sneezing and coughing.

The substantia nigra

The colour of the black matter (substantia nigra or nucleus niger) is the result of this core containing a large quantity of iron and melanin pigment. This core has been carefully studied since Parkinson's disease results from the neural degeneration of this ganglion. The nerve fibres run from it to the cerebral cortex and the corpus striatum. Outbound nerve fibres go to the thalamus. The melanin-containing nerve cells (neurons) of the nucleus niger produce a significant quantity of dopamine and thus regulate the entire circuit of motion control. In Parkinson's disease, these cells degenerate so that the inhibiting control mediated by dopamine grows weaker and weaker. This produces the symptoms of Parkinson's disease: marked trembling (tremor), rigid facial expression, slower movements and gait, and stiff muscles etc., all described in detail in the Bircher-Benner Manual No. 1. In addition to the inhibiting control of the black nucleus, the motoric movements are also controlled through inhibition by nerve cells from two other basal ganglia: through the pale core (globus pallidus) and a core below the thalamus (nucleus subthalamicus). When these fail, the control of the black core (nucleus niger) becomes predominant, which leads to the continuous, tormenting, excessive spontaneous waving movements of Huntington's disease, a congenital disease, or chorea minor if these cores are affected in the scope of the autoimmune reactions of rheumatic fever.

The black core can be viewed as one rein of the coachman, and the globus pallidus with the subthalamic nucleus as the other. If one rein is pulled too strongly, the motion disorder of Parkinson's disease results; when the other one is pulled too strongly, choreatic disorder (St. Vitus's dance) results.

The limbic system

The structures of the limbic system form a double ring around the basal ganglia and the thalamus. The limbic system is formed partly by phylogenetically old sections of the cerebral cortex (archipallium) and brain structures that are placed below the cerebral cortex. The name comes from limbus (seam), since the system is situated as a ring below the cerebrum hemispheres on both sides. This includes the hippocampus, fornix, corpus mamillare, gyrus cinguli, corpora amygdalae, front parts of the thalamus, septum pellucidum and a brain convolution at the side of the hippocampus.

To the limbic system is ascribed the processing of emotions and it is linked to all the other brain structures. Damage to the limbic system produces the following neuropsychological defects: inability to assess emotional situations, memory problems, post-traumatic stress disorders, autism, depression, phobias and narcolepsy (inadvertent sleeping during the day).

Alzheimer's disease damages the hippocampus (part of the limbic system) at an early stage, so that emotional disorders occur early on. Schizophrenia will often reveal reduced circulation in the limbic system in PET scans. Bipolar disorder is also ascribed to damage to the limbic system. Neuroleptics and sleeping pills, such as benzodiazepines (Valium, Temesta, etc.), have a manipulatory effect on the limbic system. In neurodegenerative diseases, degenerative damage to the limbic system is largely responsible for personality change.

The motor pathways

The nerve pathways for moving the body's muscles (tractus corticospinalis) cross at the level of the medulla oblongata, so that any stimulation of a left side motoneuron of the left cerebral cortex leads to a reaction in the right half of the body. The cerebral cortex contains the 'first' motoneuron (proximal motoneuron). Its long nerve extension (neurite) reaches down into the spinal cord in long pathways until it contacts a segment assigned to it (level). There the nerve extension (neurite) reaches its assigned second nerve cell (distal or second motoneuron) in the foremost lateral part (anterior horn), which may have a very long nerve pathway to the assigned muscles.

The sensitive tracks

The same course in the reverse direction is taken by sensory nerves (sensitive nerves and nerve pathways). Their first nerve cell is located in the organ or skin area that produces the sensation. Their nerve extension (neurite) reaches into the posterior horn of the spinal cord in the segment (spinal cord level) assigned to it, where it passes on its perception to a second nerve cell (second neuron). The nerve fibres of all of these second neurons run as rear strands in the rear spinal cord up to the thalamus, where they are switched and selected (as previously described) before transmitting the information to the cerebral cortex and into the conscious mind.

The hormone-producing glands of the brain

The best-known of the hormone-producing glands is the pituitary gland (hypophysis). The hypothalamus is located below the thalamic nucleus. It controls the hormone production in the body by measuring the hormone concentrations in the blood and adjusting them to the current demand. If the amount of a specific hormone to be produced is to be increased, the hypothalamus will send a substance (hormone-releasing factor) to the pituitary gland, which will cause the corresponding hormone to be produced to an increasing degree.

The anterior lobe of the hypophysis (adenohypophysis) produces the following hormones:

Thyroxine releasing hormone (TSH)
This stimulates the thyroid cells to increase production of thyroid hormones T3 and T4. If their levels (concentrations) in the blood grow too high, the hypothalamus will register the fact and reduce its stimulation again.

ACTH (adrenocorticotropic hormone)
Its excretion is regulated in the same manner. It stimulates the glandular cells of the adrenal glands to increase the production of cortisol.

FSH (follicle stimulating hormone)
This is regulated in the same manner and stimulates the production of oestrogens and the follicle maturation of the ovum, as well as the production of sperm in the male.

LH (luteinising hormone)
Causes ovulation and stimulates the production of progesterone (gestagen) for the production of the corpus luteum in the second half of the menstrual cycle. In the male, it stimulates production of the masculinising hormone testosterone, which is also relevant in the female but in a lesser concentration.

PRL (prolactin)
This stimulates the mammary gland to produce milk while at the same time inhibiting the production of sex hormones (gonadotropins).

STH or GH (somatotropin or growth hormone)
This promotes body growth as long as the epiphyseal plates remain open. It promotes the release of fatty tissue and conversion of fat into sugar. It releases the insulin-like growth factor (insulin-like growth factor IgF1).

MSH (melanocyte-stimulating hormone or melanotropin)
It stimulates the pigment-forming cells (melanocytes) to increase pigment production.

The posterior pituitary (neurohypophysis)

Its two hormones are formed in the hypothalamic nucleus and these migrate down into the posterior pituitary, which in turn releases them into the blood. These two hormones are:

ADH (antidiuretic hormone or vasopressin)
This hormone causes the integration of resorption channels (aquaporin) into the collective tubes of the kidneys, so that more water from the primary urine is absorbed back into the blood.

Oxytocin
This hormone causes the uterus to contract and milk to be excreted by the mammary glands. The relationship between mother and child is greatly deepened by it during breastfeeding. Oxytocin is also emitted during tender moments, as when caressing and singing. It produces a deep feeling of belonging and security.

The epiphysis and melatonin

The epiphysis is about 7 mm large and located at the very rear, below the corpus callosum.

It produces the hormone melatonin when it becomes dark outside. Synthetic light suppresses its production also, and this impairs sleep. It has been documented that melatonin is very important for learning and spatial memory[2]. Melatonin plays an important role in regulating the circadian rhythm and sleep. In the United States today Melatonin is sold over the counter as a sleeping pill. However, the National Institute of Aging has issued warnings about the casual use of melatonin.

The nerve cell (neuron)

Each of the approx. 100 billion nerve cells of the brain comprises a cell body with cytoplasm and a nucleus. One or several protrusions grow from this to receive the information (neurites), along with a very long protrusion that forwards the information (neurite). The protrusion can be more than one metre long. All of these protrusions contain cellular fluid deep inside, as well as mitochondria for cell respiration and a supply of energy-providing phosphates. The nerve cell and dendrites belong to the grey matter of the brain, since they have no myelin sheaths that would colour them white.

The dendrites
Dendrites have multiple branches and are able to find other nerve cells and nerve fibres with their endings, thereby amplifying the linking of information in the central nervous system. This adjustment is very important in the development of the brain in children and is retained to an advanced age. The learning of new skills, thinking, cognitive tasks and making music all promote new links. If skills are not needed, the links between the dendrites are removed. This adaptability is called brain plasticity.

The neurites

Neurites are the forwarding nerve fibres. They run through the brain and spinal cord in bundles and pathways and combine in the body into nerve roots and nerves.

The inside of the neurites is called the axon (Greek for axis). It contains the cell membranes, cytoplasm and mitochondria, and is fed from the cell body. The axon is enveloped by cells of the connective tissue of the brain (glial cells) by multiple convolutions of a myelin-containing layer, 95 % of which are made of fats, with a high content of cholesterol and polyunsaturated fatty acids that colour the neurites white. The body nerves have special cells (Schwann cells) that produce the myelin sheaths. The myelin sheath is constricted after a little less than every thousandth millimetre (nodes of Ranvier). Stimulation jumps from node to node. This increases the nerve conduction speed considerably.

The potential for action

Potassium is pumped in and sodium out at the membranes of the nerve cells, thereby producing an electrical potential of about 80 thousandth of a volt (80 mV, resting potential) at the cell membrane. When the nerve cell receives a large quantity of information from its dendrites, the potential increases until there is a discharge, and the nerve cell transmits information through its neurites.

If the nervous system is overstimulated, the resting potential increases and little is required to produce a discharge. If the resting potential is reduced, the nerve cell will react late and slowly. A high magnesium level and a high calcium level in the blood stabilise the nervous system, while low sodium or high potassium considerably increases its excitability.

The synapses

These are connections in which signals are transferred by one nerve cell to another or to muscle fibres. The complexity of the dendritic networking in the brain is extremely differentiated. A cerebellum cell, for example, will take up signals from other nerve cells through about 100,000 dendritic synapses. Transfer of the action potential via the synapses usually takes place through chemical transmitters (neurotransmitters).

There are different types of synapses: those with stimulating and those with inhibiting messenger substances.

Stimulating messenger substances

Glutamate is the most important exciting neurotransmitter of the brain and is involved in many processes, such as the controlling circuits of motor control in the basal ganglia, where Parkinson's disease and Huntington's disease result. A special glutamate receptor, the NMDA receptor, is involved in learning processes[3].

Noradrenaline is located in many synapses of nuclei of the brainstem. In the vegetative nervous system of the body, it transfers the signals of the ganglia of the sympathetic nervous system.

Adrenaline is not a neurotransmitter, by contrast. It is excreted only as a hormone by the adrenal gland and unfolds its effect at the synapses of noradrenaline throughout the organism.

Acetylcholine acts on the parasympathetic (calming) vegetative nervous system in the ganglia and at the synapses of the transfer of signals of the motoric nerves to the muscle fibres (motoric end plate).

Inhibiting messenger substances

GABA (γ-aminobutyric-acid) is the most important inhibiting messenger substance of the brain. GABA acts at the synapses of many nuclei in the brain. Members of the group of medicines of the benzodiazepines (Valium, Temesta, etc.) act at the GABA receptors of these synapses and cause a general dampening of the central nervous system in this way. They have a sedative effect, and thus reduce anxiety and muscle tension.

Glycine is an inhibiting neurotransmitter that is mostly found in the spinal cord.

Serotonin plays a role especially in the area of the brain stem and the pituitary gland. It has a certain mood-lifting effect. Depression can be alleviated by adjusting the serotonin level through medication.

The importance of the glial cells in the brain

The name 'glia' comes from Greek and means 'glue'. The supporting function of the glia cells and their fibres for the nerve cells (neurons) were recognised at an early stage. Most glial cells come from the outer layer of the germ layer (ectoderm), but the microglial cells are from the middle layer (mesoderm). As far as we know today, the glial cells not only form a supporting structure for the nerve cells, but they also provide electrical insulation with their protective envelopes. Furthermore, the glial cells are involved essentially with the substance transport and fluid exchange, and in the maintenance of the homeostasis in the brain. Additionally, they contribute to the process of information processing, storage and forwarding. Glial cells are usually smaller than nerve cells. In the posterior pituitary (neurohypophysis), specialised glial cells (pituicytes) influence transport, storage and release of the antidiuretic hormone (ADH) and the hormone oxytocin by the nerve fibres.

Most glial cells of the brain are astrocytes that resemble stars with their many protrusions. They regulate the potassium and fluid balance in the brain and the acid-base balance. They are also involved in processing of information in the brain. They contain vesicles with the stimulating neurotransmitter glutamate. Its release can activate adjacent nerve cells. If nerve fibres (axons) are injured, they form glial scars. However, this prevents new growth of the nerve fibres and thus prevents healing of paraplegia. Special astrocytes function as important conductive structures in the early development of the brain.

The oligodendroglia cells form the myelin for the electrical insulation of the nerve fibres (axons).

Microglial cells make up about 20 % of all glial cells. During brain development, they ensure the correct number of predecessor cells for the nerve cells (neurons). Then they participate in immune defence by turning into macrophages. Since antibodies cannot enter the brain across the blood-brain barrier in a healthy person, the microglial cells are responsible for the immune defence against inflammation in the brain. They also support the nerve cells in regeneration after injury[4]. Thus the microglial cells have a function similar to that of macrophages in the immune system in other tissues, since they remove the cell residues of dead nerve cells and oligodendrocytes by phagocytosis (absorption and dissolution).

It is assumed that the microglial cells are produced from predecessor cells of the blood-forming system just like the other immune cells in embryonic development. They also act as antigen-presenting cells in the brain once they are activated by a suspicious molecule. This activation is, for example, involved in the degenerative inflammation processes of multiple sclerosis. Like amoebae, they migrate to the site of the inflammation and gather there. Once they arrive there, they remove cell toxins such as hydrogen superoxide or nitrogen monoxide, dead cell substances and foreign bodies. After removing defective body tissue and foreign substances, they emit specific cytokines (such as interleukin-1, tumour necrosis factor α, interferon γ) into the space outside of the cells (extracellular space). In this way, the astrocytes increase and form glial scar tissue.

The spaces of the brain and the fluid in the brain and spinal cord

The fluid in the brain (liquor cerebrospinalis) is excreted from the two lateral cavities (lateral ventricles) made up of capillaries, a type of vasoganglions (plexus choroideus). This ensures substance transport from the blood to the brain in a highly complex manner and at the same time prevents unacceptable substances from getting from the blood to the meninges and the brain fluid (blood-brain barrier). From the lateral ventricles, the brain fluid flows into the middle third ventricle, from there into the fourth ventricle below, and from there into the thin spinal canal at the centre of the spinal cord. The brain fluid then enters the space of the web-like cerebral membrane (meningea arachnoidea) and is resorbed into the blood. The brain fluid contains only little protein in a healthy person and very few white blood corpuscles.

The blood-brain barrier

The blood-brain barrier protects the brain from pathogens, toxins and messenger substances circulating in the blood. It is a highly selective filter through which the nutrients needed by the brain are supplied, and meta bolites produced in the metabolism are discharged. This entire substance exchange is ensured by a great many ingeniously conceived transport processes.

The blood-brain barrier is only very rarely the cause of disease, but is very often stressed and damaged by it. It usually holds back medicines, so that the pharmaceutical industry has to carry out significant research to bring medicines to the desired place to affect the brain. The blood capillaries are very carefully sealed from the brain tissue by 'tight junctions'. Glial cells keep careful watch over the capillaries being sealed.

The brain's mass makes up only 2 % of the body's total mass. Its share in the nutrient demand is approx. 20 %, however. In contrast to the other organs, the brain has almost no nutrient and oxygen reserves. Nerve cells can survive for no more than three minutes without oxygen. The brain cannot handle interferences with the acid-base balance (pH-deviations). Fluctuations of the potassium content must not reach the brain any more than should the messenger substances of the synapses (neurotransmitters) that circulate in the blood vessels. The great impermeability of the blood-brain barrier to pathogens, antibodies and white blood corpuscles (leukocytes) circulating in the blood makes them an immunological barrier so that the cells of the microglia must take over the function of the immune defence.

The high energy demand of the brain produces an above-average amount of metabolites that must be discharged through the blood-brain barrier.

The complex functions of the brain are bound to highly sensitive electrochemical and biochemical processes that can only run in a constant inner environment, homeostasis, usually without interference. Changes to the blood-brain barrier cause changes to the condition of the central nervous system, which in turn may cause function impairment or diseases of the central nervous system. Accordingly, a number of neurological diseases are connected to changes to the blood-brain barrier.

The brain is permeated by more than 100 billion capillaries, the total length of which has been calculated to be approx. 600 km[5]. The cerebral cortex contains 300 to 800 capillary cross sections per mm^2. The total area of the blood vessels in the brain is estimated at 12 to 20[6,7], making the sealing of this large area of capillaries extremely difficult. The cells that form the capillary walls (endothelial cells) are thin. In contrast to the capil-laries in the remaining part of the body, they are sealed by being attached to each other (tight junctions). The astrocytes of the macroglia monitor the formation and sealing of the endothelial cells and place complex end feet on the capillary walls for sealing purposes. Highly specialised cells of the microglia (pericytes) regulate cell division of the endothelial cells in the capillary walls. They secrete the substance actin, with which they change the diameter of the capillaries and thus regulate the blood pressure in the brain vessels. These pericytes are also able to convert to macrophages, eliminate foreign and toxic substances, and present antigens to the immune cells[8,9,10,11].

Transport through the blood-brain barrier
The membranes of the blood-brain barrier contain fat (lipophilic). Nevertheless, tiny molecules (less than 0.52 nm^2) can diffuse through the blood-brain barrier. This is made possible by a very small kink of a membrane molecule producing a tiny gap that goes through the membrane with the molecule[12,13,14].

Fat-soluble (lipophilic) substances generally pass most easily through the plasma membranes of cells made of fatty acids. Nevertheless, in patients six years old and older, 98 % of the medicines that are of small, fat-soluble molecules and etheric oils are no longer able to enter the brain.

Small molecules with a polar charge, such as the water molecule, can only diffuse through the wall of the capillaries within very strict limits through the hydrophobic kinks. Nevertheless, large amounts of water can pass the blood-brain barrier to the brain. For this purpose the membranes contain hydrophilic (water-soluble) protein molecules (aquaporins, canal proteins). Glycerine and urea molecules can also pass through such canal proteins.

There is a special transport system for the transport of glucose and amino acids to the brain in the capillary membrane (GLUT-1 transporter). Other transport systems (MCT-1 und 2) can transport organic acids, such as lactic acid, pyruvic acid (pyruvate), mevalonate, butyrates and acetate. There are special transport systems for nutrients, vitamins, hormones, trace elements and folic acid as well.

There are special transport systems for various larger molecules that consume energy. Selected large molecules, such as the iron-containing transferrin or the LDL cholesterol, which is very important for the brain, are fed through the membrane of the capillaries by small vesicles (vesicular transport) and include insulin and other peptide hormones and cytokines for the immune defence. Other selected peptides (short-chained proteins) and proteins (larger protein molecules) are fed through the membrane because of their positive charge (cationic transport)[15].

Many neurodegenerative diseases, but also diabetes, considerably impair the blood-brain barrier. Certain pathogens can pass this barrier as well, including the HI and other viruses and bacteria, such as Neisseria meningitidis or the cholera bacterium (Vibrio cholerae)[16].

The behaviour of the blood-brain barrier in substance transport into and out of the brain

Extremely fat-soluble, unpolar substances (solvents) and chlorinated hydrocarbons pass unhindered through the lipid-containing membranes of the blood-brain barrier into the brain. Other substances, such as many nutrients (amino acids, sugar, vitamins) can only pass the blood-brain barrier using active and passive transport systems. All of the cell types named for the blood-brain barrier form a functional system that is also called a 'neurovascular unit'. This ensures unhindered transport of vital nutrients from the blood, removal of the degradation products of the metabolism from the brain into the blood, and the recognition and elimination of harmful foreign substances or toxins if these are not fat-soluble. The blood-brain barrier also has specific substance transport systems for this purpose.

Larger molecule complexes, viruses and small particles are transported in small vesicles that are fed through the membrane in a complex manner. Some of these transport systems are only active in one direction. One is the P-glycoprotein system in the membrane of the capillary walls. This binds foreign and hazardous substances to its receptor (PgP receptor) and feeds foreign and hazardous substances out of the brain into the blood. The blood-brain barrier can also feed neurologically and immunologically active substances such as nitric oxide (NO), prostaglandins and cytokines (messenger substances from immune cells) out of the brain into the blood.

On the other hand, the blood-brain barrier is less tight in the liquor cavities (brain ventricles) and the olfactory brain, so that acti- vating messenger substances (cytokines such as the interleukins IL1-α, IL1-β, β IL-6, TNF-α and interferon IFN-γ) from inflammations and suppurative foci of the body, the intestine or from abscesses of tooth roots can enter the brain from the body. These activate the immune system of the microglia and are therefore largely responsible for the chronic inflammatory processes in the brain that cause multiple sclerosis and the other neurodegenerative diseases[17].

Various studies also showed that 12 different interleukins, when present in abundance in the body, can cross the blood-brain barrier and thus get from the blood into the brain. It has been documented that various cytokines, including IL1-α, IL1-β, TNF-α and IFN-γ, can enter the brain if they are highly concentrated in the blood. This has led to the conclusion that there must be specific transport systems for these cytokines in the membrane of the endothelial cells of the capillaries of the brain[18].

The effect of alcohol consumption on the blood-brain barrier

Alcohol consumption damages the blood-brain barrier. It is a main risk factor for inflammatory diseases of the nervous system and for susceptibility towards bacterial infections[19, 20, 21]. Damage to the blood-brain barrier from alcohol is considered to be an essential influence for the development of some neurodegenerative diseases[22]. Damage to the blood-brain barrier is documented by neuropathological examinations of alcoholics as well as in animal experiments[23]. In the animal experiment, it has been found that the enzyme myosin light-chain kinase (MLCK) that is activated by alcohol consumption causes phosphorylation of several tight junctions or cytoskeletal proteins in the endothelium, where the integrity of the blood-brain barrier is impaired[24]. Alcohol consumption leads to significant oxidative stress that additionally damages the blood-brain barrier[25]. It is not the alcohol as such, but its degradation products (metabolites) that activate the myosin light-chain enzyme (MLCK) in the endothelial cells of the capillary walls. The damage to the blood-brain barrier from consumption of alcohol assists the ingression of white blood corpuscles (leucocytes) into the brain, which facilitates inflammatory processes in the brain such as the ones relevant for multiple sclerosis[22].

The effect of smoking on the blood-brain barrier
It has been shown in several studies that smokers have a much higher risk of developing dementia from Alzheimer's disease than non-smokers[26]. Extended administration of nicotine to test animals changed the function and structure of the blood-brain barrier[27]. In epidemiological studies, a much higher risk of bacterial meningitis has been documented for smokers[28].

The effect of electromagnetic radiation on the human brain and the blood-brain barrier
The harmful effect of the pulsed high-frequency radiation from mobile phones, in the mega- to gigahertz range, have been scientifically documented[29]. This applies similarly to the radiation from mobile house phones, wireless connections on computers, WLAN and remote controls. There is no consensus yet about the harm caused by this radiation in a lower energy range. High energy density of electromagnetic radiation has been shown to cause considerable heating in the affected body tissue. In the skull, this heat can impair the blood-brain barrier and make it more permeable[30].

The power required for a 15-minute call by mobile phone heats the brain much less than a hot bath, though heating from the bath causes no damage[27]. The Swedish university in Lund proved that the blood-brain barrier, as well as the neurons of the brain, can be damaged even without the effect of heating from a mobile phone's radiation[31, 32, 33, 34].

Physics differentiates between electromagnetic waves and scalar waves. Scalar waves are also used in mobile phones. They can pass through concrete walls like jackhammers and reach even a distant child's bedroom, the iron-reinforced basement in houses and the underground floors and parking garages of supermarkets and other shopping centres.

Physics differentiates thus between transverse waves (Hertz) and scalar waves (Tesla). Transverse waves cannot enter metal grids or cages (Faraday cage). They can hardly pass through reinforced concrete walls and ceilings, and cannot enter cars or elevators at all. One hundred years ago, the physician Tesla discovered a wave type that cannot be held back by anything and that passes through everything: the scalar wave. This longitudinal wave is aligned lengthwise and forms wave vortexes. Today's mobile phones work mainly with scalar waves.

The risk of damage is that our biological system works with scalar waves as well, e.g. the morphogenetic fields that affect the differentiation of body forms on the basis of the genetic material. Sunlight reaches us as a transverse wave and is converted into scalar waves (standing light wave equals photon) when entering the biological system. As we have seen, the sunlight is greatly amplified according to the LASER principle and saved in the genetic substance of the cells.

The frequency pattern of the spontaneous brain activity in the electroencephalogram corresponds to that of sunlight. The human brain thus works with scalar waves; brain currents are disastrously cycled within the same scalar wave frequency window as the scalar waves of mobile phones[35].

The myelin marrow sheaths – a sensitive substance

Myelin is a biomembrane that spirally envelops the nerve strands (axons). It is made of up to 70 % fats (lipids) and 30 % protein. Because of the high fat content, the fast-conducting nerve pathways appear white and consequently form the white substance in the brain. The fast-conducting nerve fibres in the body are also enveloped by myelin sheaths.

In the brain, myelin is formed by the cells of the microglia (oligodendrocytes); in the nerves in the body, however, myelin is formed by Schwann cells. Myelin is complex in its structure: myelin fats are 25 % cholesterol, 20 % galactocerebroside, 5 % galacto-sulfatide and 50 % mainly phosphatidylethanolamine and lecithin. The proteins are myelin basic protein (MBP), proteolipid protein (PLP/DM20), myelin-associated glycoprotein (MAG) and connexin (CX32). In addition, myelin oligodendrocyte glycoprotein (MOG) appears in the brain, and protein zero (P0, MPZ) and peripheral myelin protein-22 (PMP-22) are found in the nerves of the body. Proteolipid protein (PLP), also called lipophilin, is important for stabilisation of the marrow sheaths.

Congenital diseases with defective myelin formation, called leukodystrophies, are rare.

Demyelinating diseases

Demyelinating diseases occur because of damage to the myelin sheaths which eventually destroys the nerve fibre running at their centre. They can also be described as 'de-marrowing' diseases.

Multiple sclerosis is by far the most common of these diseases. Other rare diseases are acute disseminated encephalomyelitis (ADEM), acute motoric axonal neuropathy, balo disease, chronically inflammatory demyelinating polyneuropathy, funicular myelosis, Miller-Fisher syndrome, transverse myelitis and neuromyelitis optica (Devic's syndrome).

Remyelination

The oligodendrocytes of the microglia of the brain are able to repair the myelin sheaths. This regeneration capacity is extremely effective in the healthy brain. The repaired myelin sheaths are much thinner. With multiple sclerosis, however, remyelination is strongly impaired because of autoimmune processes, so that it is insufficient for healing.

At present, many research centres are seeking to understand why remyelination is not successful in multiple sclerosis. Apparently the stem cells of the oligodendrocytes do not mature. Messenger substances from inflammation cells (cytokines) inhibit maturation of the oligodendrocytes from their preliminary stages. The tumour necrosis factors 2 and α play key roles in this[30]. Chemokines conduct the oligodendrocytes to the place of degenerated myelin and promote maturing of the oligodendrocytes. In multiple sclerosis, chemokine CXCL12 is strongly reduced. Residues of degenerated myelin also are supposed to activate the cell receptor LINGO1, which prevents remyelination and maturation of oligodendrocytes[32]. With increasing age, remyelination declines. It is presumed that the genes responsible for this are reduced in their activity[37]. Certain growth factors promote remyelination, such as the factor EGF and others[32]. Certain cell receptors (toll-like receptors) have also been found that inhibit maturation of the oligodendrocytes and thus remyelination[38].

Many other factors and influences are being researched. In multiple sclerosis, it has been documented that remyelination initially is still very efficient but fails as the disease progresses chronically[39]. Researchers are trying to find medicines to block the receptors Notch-1, Wnt and LINGO1, which inhibit cell maturation. Multiple sclerosis is described in Bircher-Benner manual no. 1 for patients with multiple sclerosis, Parkinson's disease and other neurodegenerative diseases.

Diseases from storage of degenerative proteins

The TAU proteins

The name is derived from the Greek letter TAU.
These are structural proteins that have been changed in their molecule structure by phosphorylation so that their task of being integrated in the microtubules of the cell skeleton can no longer be met. They are therefore stored in the nerve cells (neurons) of the brain, where they form twisted fibres (twisted fibrils). Nine of such diseases, called tauopathies, have been so far identified.

The fibrils destroy the neurons entirely, resulting in a slow death to the brain.
By far the best known of the tauopathies is Alzheimer's disease. It also presents intense depositing of beta amyloids in the inter-cell substance, the basic substance of the brain. Alzheimer's disease is not a genetic disease. Causative connections have been documented in relation to widespread poor nutrition with too many animal products, to various environmental pollutants and to pulsed high-frequency radiation from mobile phones.

Amyloidosis

Amyloidosis means enrichment of abnormally changed proteins in the inter-cell substances, the basic substance of the soft connective tissue that runs through the entire body and ensures all exchanges of substances between the blood capillaries and the cells. The degenerative change renders the proteins insoluble in water. They are therefore present in the form of small fibres, called fibrils. They are called β-fibrils. These pathological deposits are caused by a pathologically changed metabolism resulting from widespread poor nutrition. The name of amyloid was given because these deposits look similar to starch under the microscope.

Amyloidosis is based on an interference in the folding of a usually soluble protein[40]. Many years of poor nutrition and several diseases may cause amyloidosis through impaired metabolism ecology, i.e. overproduction, missing or reduced breaking down or impaired excretion of certain proteins. The proteins are in a dissolved form in the blood vessels and capillaries. If their concentration increases, they will get into the inter-cell substance of the surrounding tissues and are attacked by enzymes. The combination of the resulting amino acid chains in the area of the β folding sheet structures β forms insoluble complexes in the form of microscopically small fibres (fibrils). These fibrils are resistant to being absorbed into macrophages (phagocytosis and proteolysis by macrophages), and therefore can no longer be broken down.

In primary amyloidosis, there is no underlying disease to be found. These are rare and sometimes occur repeatedly in one family. Secondary amyloidosis are by far the most common ones. There is an underlying disease as the cause, such as chronic inflammation, chronic infection, tumours of the lymphatic system or long dialysis treatment.

Many elderly persons suffer from old-age amyloidosis, deposits in particular in the heart or brain, in the form of β-amyloid in the inter-cell substance, as is the case in Alzheimer's disease. This is also called AS-amyloidosis, or senile amyloidosis. As mentioned before, the cause lies in widespread poor nutrition and the resulting considerable impairment of the metabolism. Amyloid deposits cause all kinds of function impairment in the brain and nerves, leading up to Alzheimer's dementia. There often are painful sensory or movement impairment in the nerves of the body (the peripheral neuropathy). If the vegetative nervous system is affected, the blood pressure will fall while the patient is standing (orthostatic weakness), weight loss from an early feeling of saturation due to reduced emptying of the stomach, erectile problems, impaired intestinal peristaltic with flatulence, stomach ache and irregular passing of stool. This book treats only the effects of amyloidosis on the central and peripheral nervous systems. The effects of amyloidosis on the heart and the blood vessels are described in Bircher-Benner manual no. 19 for high blood pressure, patients with cardiac diseases and arteriosclerosis.

The effect of nutrition on the central nervous system

Two kinds of food energy

Physicists are aware of two types of energy: the orderly and the chaotic. Orderly energy saves information. Chaotic energy cannot save anything. Heat energy (calories) is chaotic energy. Sunlight is the most highly ordered form of energy. Its information is in a way similar to a large symphony. Listening to a symphony does not produce heat, but it provides information: it is a highly orderly sound structure that triggers precise sensations and feelings. With its complex oscillations, sunlight conveys and orders the genetically specified information that is needed for the growth, differentiation and regeneration of all life on earth.

One green leaf contains about one million chlorophyll funnels. At the base of each funnel, there are two chlorophyll α molecules each. The funnel reflects the incoming light into the base, where two chlorophyll α molecules enter into a maximum resonance, synchronised with the oscillations of the solar radiation (coherence). They convert the energy from this resonance into UV light, which makes them light up (invisibly to our eyes). This light flows through the entire plant body, all the way to the roots and the tips of the roots[41,42]. All living cells store UV light in their molecules, especially in the ring-shaped molecules.

The double helix of the genetic material in the cell cores stores by far the most light. The double helix (DNA) can coil to the right or left and can form protrusions shaped like clover leaves, radiating specific UV light spectrums[43]. The double helix of the DNA serves as a cavity resonator for the rhythmic LASER amplification of UV-light in our cells[44]. For a LASER to begin to work, it must receive a certain amount of energy. Bio-physicians call this minimum energy supply the LASER threshold. In their experiments, researchers of the International Academy for Biophoton Research measured the LASER threshold in plant tissues[43].

Just like plants, human and animal cells store UV-l-light in their DNA[45,40]. We lack the ability to photosynthesise, however, and direct application of sunlight to the skin is far from enough to keep our LASER light storage above the LASER threshold.

The plant's cell stores the photons from sunlight in incredible quantity. It could be shown that the ultra-weak cell radiation[41] is nothing but a leakage radiation, a tiny leak of the UV-light through the cell membrane. Measurements showed that LASER amplification of the light is 104 times stronger in the DNA than that provided by technical LASER devices. The inside of the cells thus represents an incredible light space.

Our photon storage must be fed daily with a sufficient amount of vital photon-containing foods, i.e. fresh vegetable foods[46,47,48].

The transmission of the information of the vital foods from photosynthesis to our organism takes place by coherence. This means that our own sensation of life, life energy and life information is renewed and reordered again and again in the roughly 50 trillion cells of our body by entering into a shared resonance with the oscillation patterns of sunlight on the transfer of the photons.

Energy inside the cell is very different from that of a non-living nature. Biophysicists call the inside of the cell a dissipative system. Russian-Belgian researcher Ilya Prigogine received a Nobel prize for his work on this.

Intense photon storage removes the energy inside the cell so far from the thermodynamic balance that the second law of thermodynamics no longer applies. This causes the chaos principle to morph into an ordering coherence principle[49].

If fresh raw foods are missing from our nutrition, the photon content in our cells will decline. The light content will fall until it drops below the LASER threshold. The cells partially revert from the principle of order (coherence principle of Prigogine[49]) to the chaos principle of thermodynamics and degenerate.

We consider disease a loss of order, a loss of ordered information. The programme of life enters into disorder and the lack of fresh, raw nutrition makes reordering impossible. Numerous experiments which were conducted among others at the University of Novosibirsk[50] show that the complex processes of biochemistry in our cells are controlled by information. If there is a lack of fresh, raw nutrition, this information will no longer be continually renewed and ordered. Thus the complex biochemical processes of our cells will be thrown into disarray. This is why fresh, raw plant food is important for its energy: it renews and strengthens the ordering resonance in the biological system.

The basic regulation system of the soft connective tissue in the central nervous system

All cells of the body's organs are embedded in the basic substance of the soft connective tissue that runs through all organs and structures. It is made up of a molecular network (matrix) of sugar-protein molecules called proteoglycans. The blood capillaries run through the basic substance, including the nerve endings of the vegetative nervous system. Outside of the central nervous system, the capillaries leak deliberately. This permits nutrients and hormones to leave them freely. They reach the cells through the network of proteoglycans, which serves as a molecular screen and information conduction system. Pathogens and toxins are drained from the matrix through the complex system of lymph vessels and cleaned in the lymph nodes. The cleansed lymph is returned into the venous blood.

We have seen that autoimmune processes of an unhealthy milieu in the intestine and a degenerated intestinal flora are stimulated because the immune cells are only able to acquire a defective immune competence under such conditions. The defective immune competence does not enable them to distinguish between external and internal correctly.

The situation in the brain is very different from that in the body. The capillary loops, which are particularly tight here since an especially large amount of oxygen and food is necessary, are sealed by the blood-brain barrier, as explained above. The neurons need an entirely different milieu than do the body cells, a milieu that is regulated and kept constant by the glial cells, particularly the astrocytes and the complex system of the transport cannels of the blood-brain barrier.

We have seen that, on the one hand, the oligodendroglial cells of the connective-tissue-like microglia protect and envelop the nerve fibres, the axons, and that, on the other hand, they take over the development and function of the immune system in the brain by converting into antigen-presenting cells and macrophages that move through the matrix of the brain like amoeba to remove intruding germs and toxins. We have also seen that the oligodendroglial cells of the microglia can repair injury to the myelin sheaths, but that this ability to regenerate the myelin (and thus the marrow sheaths of the fast-conducting nerve fibres) is exhausted in, for example, multiple sclerosis due to the long-term autoimmune inflammation.

We have seen that abnormal degenerated proteins (β-amyloids) are deposited in the matrix of the brain tissue if the metabolic economy is not ensured and that these deposits of β-amyloids in the basic system of the connective tissue of the brain are one of the central causes of dementia from Alzheimer's disease. We have also seen how certain proteins that are supposed to help stabilise the cell membranes (cytoskeleton) change abnormally under the same prerequisites, making them phosphorylated. Instead of accomplishing their tasks, they become twisted fibrils that destroy the nerve cells of the brain.

Food economy and food energy play a key role in keeping the matrix and the basic regulation system with the network of proteoglycans beyond the blood-brain barrier healthy, both in the body and in the central nervous system. We will see below that the depositing of toxic heavy metals, oxidative stress from an unnatural lifestyle, poor nutrition and electromagnetic radiation damage not only the proper function of the blood-brain barrier, but also the basic regulation system of the brain and the neurons themselves, as well as the myelin sheaths, directly and severely, so that the immune system of the brain spins out of control and attacks the damaged degenerating tissue and the myelin sheaths through an autoimmune reaction that destroys the marrow sheaths and thus causes multiple sclerosis. An autoimmune reaction that destroys the marrow sheaths, causing multiple sclerosis, that leads to Parkinson's disease through deposits of alpha-synuclein in the substantia nigra, and to Alzheimer's through degenerative oxidative phosphorylation of the TAU proteins and deposits of β-amyloid in the matrix. The key to understanding the causes of this and other neurodegenerative diseases is to be found here. It is the key to a treatment that is particularly effective for this disease and that is described in this book.

Oxidative stress at the centre of the causes of neurodegenerative diseases

Unsuitable nutrition, irritants, environmental stress, a disorderly lifestyle, ionising, and electromagnetic and UV radiation all cause the organism to suffer from oxidative stress. This results in a metabolic situation in which in the physiological context a totally excessive amount of reactive oxygen compounds (R.O.S., or reactive oxygen species) occurs. These highly reactive oxidising substances are molecules with at least one unsaturated electron pair, which makes them particularly reactive. They are produced in the mitochondria, the 'power plants' of the cells that break down glucose through electron transfer and the enzyme cytochrome P 450-oxidase.

This produces the superoxide anion radical O_2^-, hydrogen peroxide (H_2O_2) and the hydroxyl radical (OH*) or nitroxygen (NO*).

Healthy cells can neutralise these highly reactive oxygen compounds with neutralising substances that they keep ready for this purpose. The most important antioxidative substance provided by the body is glutathione, a peptide that it produces from the three amino acids glutamic acid, cysteine and glycine. Other important antioxidants are ubiquinone (of coenzyme Q10), vitamins A, C and E, selenium and many secondary plant substances from vegetable food.

In the case of oxidative stress in the metabolism, these reserves will have been depleted, and oxidised glutathione can then no longer be returned to its active, reduced form sufficiently, since the enzyme glutathione reductase is depleted, as well as other detoxification enzymes such as peroxide dismutase and catalase. The highly reactive oxidants (R.O.S.) thus remain in the metabolism, where they can damage large molecules (macro molecules) inside and outside the cells.

This has dangerous consequences. The unsaturated fatty acids of the cell membranes are oxidised *(lipid peroxidation)*, and this causes the destruction of the mitochondria, the power plants in the cells, exhausting the cells and requiring them to expend much more energy in order to maintain their electrical membrane potentials. Additionally, the lipid-containing myelin sheaths of the fast-conducting nerve fibres in the brain and the spinal cord and in the nerves outside of the central nervous system are damaged by lipid peroxidation. Additionally, there will be further damage to proteins *(protein peroxidation)* and the hereditary material *(DNA peroxidation)*, which causes the DNA molecules of the hereditary material to split (genetic mutations) and may lead to the conversion of healthy cells into tumour or cancer cells.

This is a premature ageing process, which significantly impairs life expectancy[51,52,53]. Glucose metabolism (in the respiratory chain of the mitochondria) produces water as its end product. In about 2 % of the cases errors occur so that, for example, an oxygen atom will connect to one instead of two hydrogen atoms. This will always create a highly reactive fission product of water: the hydroxyl radical (OH*). This *free radical* is very reactive since the oxygen atom of the OH* radical is actively searching for an additional electron from another molecule. Other radicals include nitric oxide (NO*), the chloride radical (Cl*), the bromide radical (Br*).

The importance of the free radicals is currently the object of much scientific interest in connection with research into the causes of various neurodegenerative diseases, such as Alzheimer's disease (AD), multiple sclerosis (MS), amyotrophic lateral sclerosis ALS), Huntington's disease and Parkinson's disease. Many studies suggest the destruction of the brain stem ganglions by free radicals as a cause of these increasingly common diseases. Multiple sclerosis shows indications of damage to the myelin sheaths from free radicals, so that the immune system reacts against the oxidised lipids. The same happens in diabetic neuropathy[54].

It is accepted among scientists today[55] that oxidative stress holds a key position among the causes of neurodegenerative diseases. The process starts with the oxidation of proteins and enzymes, which change their spatial structure (tertiary structure) because of their oxidation and form an insoluble beta folding sheet structure that is then deposited in the brain in the form of aggregates – LEWY bodies in Parkinson's disease and β-amyloid plaques in Alzheimer's disease – where they destroy the nerve cells.

Usually, the correct folding of the protein is achieved by using special protein complexes (chaperones). It is suspected that these cha-peperone complexes are changed by oxidative and nitrosative stress, so that they can no longer perform their function in the production of a correct three-dimensional structure of the proteins. The insoluble degenerative proteins deposited inside and outside the nerve cells cause programmed cell death (apoptosis). Cell death is caused by excessive excretion of the activating neurotransmitter glutamate. Glutamate activates a receptor in the cell membranes (NMDA receptor) that trips a permanent calcium flow into the nerve cells. This activates an enzyme NO-synthase), which causes the nitric oxide radical (NO*) to form. In the mitochondria, excess calcium inhibits cell respiration. This causes massive formation of free radicals (R.O.S.). The radical NO* is further oxidised into the highly reactive peroxynitrite, massively damaging the membranes by lipid peroxidation together with the other free radicals (R.O.S.). This releases the substance cytochrome C, which starts the biologically determined cascade of cell destruction (apoptosis). The brain has a cell-preserving substance that protects the nerve cells from destruction by apoptosis. In this way, they would be protected from healthy adjacent cells. Since the adjacent cells are also attacked, this protection factor is missing and cell death spreads through the tissue of the brain.

The influence of environmental stress from pollutants as the cause of neuro-generative diseases

Recent research has shown the direct toxic effects of many chemicals that in the brain lead to neurodegenerative diseases in the long term. For example, even low concentrations of mould as well as chemicals in the domestic environment may cause behavioural and memory problems[56]. This effect involves the glial cells, which are immunologically active, form part of the blood-brain barrier and are in direct, close contact with the nerve fibres.

The neurotoxic effect of mercury

This metal, which is a liquid at room temperature, is one of the most toxic chemical elements on our planet. Nevertheless, it has been introduced into the teeth of many millions of people in the last 160 years in the form of amalgam fillings. It is available as a salt in mono- and bivalent forms (Hg^+, Hg^{++}). Organic mercury compounds are formed from this as well, in particular the highly toxic methylmercury ($CH_3·Hg^+$). Tooth amalgams contain more than 50 % mercury, as well as silver, copper and tin; these metals too are neurotoxic. In 2006, approx. 2000 tons of pure mercury were processed into tooth amalgams and used in dental fillings[57].

It is characteristic of the mercury in amalgam fillings that it evaporates constantly, so that concentrations of up to 52 µg/m³ air have been measured in the mouth[58]. The amount of evaporation depends on the number of amalgam fillings and the pressure exerted when chewing[59]. In the brains of people with amalgam fillings, concentrations of mercury two to twelve times higher have been measured than those in the amalgam-free control group[60]. Amalgam is transferred from the mother to the unborn child. Several studies showed that the mercury content in the brains of infants who died of sudden infant death correlated with the number of amalgam fillings of the mothers[61]. This meets the toxicological criterion of the dosage effect principle.

Under the microscope, the highly toxic effect of mercury on the nerves can be observed and filmed directly. Even a concentration of 0.1 µMol/litre results in rapid degeneration of the nerve fibre (axon). A concentration of 0,18 µg Hg/l leads to a deposit of β-amyloid and a protein hyperphosphorylation by binding phosphorus to the TAU-protein, both of which are present in Alzheimer's disease[62]. This shows the extreme neurotoxicity of even very small doses of mercury – much lower concentrations than those measured in the organs of amalgam carriers. Additionally, these tests only used the ionised mercury Hg^{++}, rather than the much more toxic elementary mercury gas $H°$, which passes the blood-brain barrier unhindered.

The gaseous mercury is ionised in the cells to become Hg^{++}. It then connects to the hydrogen sulphide groups of the proteins of organic substances such as hormones, neurotransmitters, peptides and enzymes. The mercury also inhibits the transport of calcium, sodium and potassium in the cell membranes, since it blocks their transport systems.

Additionally, mercury salts in the organism connect to methyl groups ($Hg-CH_3$). Methylated mercury is fat-soluble. Therefore, it collects in the myelin sheaths of the brain, the spinal cord and the nerve sheaths. This impairs functions of the brain and spinal cord and leads to signs of peripheral polyneuropathy (nerve damage) such as tri, impaired sensation and paralysis. Additionally, methylmercury causes the release of free radicals (R.O.S.) in the mitochondria of all cells. Through increasing oxidative and nitrosative stress, this causes nerve cells to die (apoptosis).

Mercury impairs the immune system severely and causes the release of cytokines (cell messenger substances) that trigger chronic inflammatory processes and provoke allergies. Mercury causes autoimmune diseases[63] and damages the dopaminergic D2-receptors of the basal ganglia of the brain, which in turn causes the symptoms of Parkinson's disease. Mercury also causes allergic diseases of the IV-type, such as hives (urticaria) and generalised eczema (neurodermatitis). In children, the appearance of a fully developed form of Feer's disease (acrodynia, Pink disease) also occurs demonstrating all the symptoms of an allergic reaction to mercury together with marked psychical and dermatological symptoms in the children.

Hair analysis best reflects the mercury deposits in the body tissues. Even mercury concentrations of 10 – 20 µg/g in the hair and 50 µg mercury/litre in the blood will cause mental and motoric retardation (development disorder of the brain). Mercury is suspected of causing autism. The mercury stress of the mother (amalgams) during pregnancy is decisive in this. A mercury content of 10 µg/g hair is deemed a risk factor for development disorders of the brain in children[64]. Methylmercury may cause developmental disorders even in the embryo[65].

Alzheimer's dementia has increased considerably in Western industrialised countries since 1970. There are significant indications of connections between the poisoning of individuals with mercury and the increase in Alzheimer's disease[66, 67].

Organic tin compounds and neurodegeneration

Organically bound tin has an antibiotic effect. Therefore, it is used to refine textiles to reduce the smell of sweat that is caused by bacterial degradation. In particular it is applied to all sports textiles. In 2000, Greenpeace purchased sports jerseys from almost all the main sports goods producers and had them examined for their content of organic tin compounds. The PVC prints of the jerseys contained up to 10.2 mg organic tin compounds per kg fabric. These were monobutyltin, dibutyltin and tributyltin.

Organic tin compounds dissolve in fat so that they can enter the brain through the blood-brain barrier unhindered. Like lead, they block cell respiration in the mitochondria of all cells. The more carbon residues are bound to a tin atom, the higher their toxicity. Triphenyltin, trimethyltin and tributyltin may cause severe poisoning even merely on skin contact[68]. Tributyltin is one of the most dangerous and toxic substances that has ever been synthetically produced and spread in the environment, according to a joint press release of the WHO and Greenpeace in 2003.

Tin poisoning results in symptoms of hyperactivity, insomnia, lack of appetite, and, later in life, general cramps and mental confusion. Trimethyltin may cause destruction of nerve cells of the brain through apoptosis. Trimethyltin causes an oedema (collection of water) in the brain and the spinal cord. This was shown in

France in 1956 in a mass poisoning caused by an antiseptic (disinfectant) called 'Salinon' that killed more than 100 persons[69]. Tributyltin does not degrade well. In the animal experiment, it caused sustained chronic damage to the liver and bile ducts and to the immune system, with acute and chronic inflammation of the pancreas (pancreatitis) cancer and malformations (teratogenic effect) and hormone-like effects on the sexual organs and the sexual characteristics, even at very low doses[70].

Organic tin compounds release the interleukins IL1-α, IL-6, TNF-a in the brain. This leads to inflammation and degeneration, which attacks the hippocampus in particular. The hippocampus is decisive for memory and learning[71].

In humans suffering from organic tin poisoning, the nerve, glial and endothelial cells are unprotected from other chemicals, so that patients will suffer from intolerance to many chemical odours and vapours in addition to the toxic effect of the tin (multiple chemical sensitivity, MCS).

Organic tin compounds were used in the coats of paint on ship hulls to prevent algae and mussels attaching to them. They are so toxic that they have caused the mass death of fish, crustaceans and mussels. These paints were finally prohibited in 2003.

Chlorine and neurodegenerative diseases

Gaseous chlorine is highly toxic to the brain and nervous system. Nevertheless, it is still sold freely in cleaning agents and disinfectants for households in any number of drug stores. Javelle water is an aqueous solution of potassium or sodium chlorite. It has a strongly oxidising and corrosive effect. Javelle water should no longer be used at all. It is neurotoxic[72]. It is suspected that this is due to the hypochlorites, such as they are also used in swimming pools, which break down into elementary chlorine, hydrogen chloride, chlorine dioxide and oxygen even if heated only slightly.

The elementary chlorine gas that gives the swimming pool and cleaning agents their typical smell penetrates the blood-brain barrier unhindered and develops its neurotoxic effect in the brain. The following neurological symptoms indicate this: general oversensitivity to any chemical and its fumes, (multiple chemical sensitivity, or MCS syndrome), excessive pain in the arms and legs (hyperaesthesia and hyperpathia) with simultaneous reduced sensitivity to touch in the arms and legs, muscle weakness, reduced reflexes, melancholy and reduced mental and emotional resilience (Benton test). The ability to concentrate and to pay attention while under stress are especially affected.

These symptoms show that chlorine gas attacks the brain (toxic encephalopathy) as well as the peripheral nerves (polyneuropathy). From a neuropsychological point of view, this suggests a reduced 'working memory', the capacity for short-term information processing. This is caused by damage to the prefrontal cerebral cortex (frontal lobes) of the hippocampus, the limbic system and the brain stem. The positron-emission tomography (PET) showed reduced glucose turnover in parts of the cerebral cortex. Additionally, the affected patients often contracted cardiovascular diseases and Alzheimer's dementia at a young age and did not live beyond the age of 45 or 50[73].

The neurotoxic effect of volatile organic hydrocarbons

House painters, car painters and mechanics, carpenters and people who work in related industries are particularly exposed to paint components and solvents.

It has been documented that even very small concentrations (in the microgram range) can cause neurotoxic damage over the years, which leads to a reduced ability to focus, fatigue and constant nausea[73, 74, 75]. Professional use of mixes of organic solvents causes severe neurotoxic damage at much lower concentrations[76].

It is important to note that the indicated MAK limits are politically negotiated values. Some of them are by a factor of 1000 greater than the scientifically determined references. In the hazardous substance mixtures, the individual references must be totalled in order to determine their toxicity[73].

Buildings treated with solvent-containing glazings and wood-protection agents may emit neurotoxic solvent vapours for a long time. If they produce disease symptoms (toxic encephalopathy), this is called 'Sick-Building Syndrome'[77]. The background stress on the population from vapours deriving from volatile organic solvents (VOC) is 300 μg/m^3, while the effect threshold for chronic stress is much lower, at 200–300 μg/m^{3,78}. Many widespread general complaints, such as fatigue, headache, sleeping disorders and lack of the ability to concentrate may have their cause in this background stress from solvent-containing paints and varnishes in rooms.

Pesticides and neurodegenerative diseases

Epidemiological studies have shown that the neurotoxicity of organic phosphorus pesticides is particularly relevant as the cause of chronic neurodegenerative diseases. Organophosphates were developed as chemical weapons by chemists of the arms industry in the early 20th century. Today, they are marketed as insecticides for agriculture, under the names chlorpyrifos, thiodicarb, parathion, fenamiphos, azinphos-methyl and methamidophos. The toxic basic substance is an organic phosphoric acid ester.

These nerve toxins cause the following symptoms: oversensitivity of the skin to light, reddening of the skin, irritation of the eyes, acute problems with breathing, choking seizures (particularly in the evening), vertigo, paralysis of the arms and legs, rheumatism-like muscle pain (myalgia), growth impairment of the nails of the fingers and toes, tremor, hearing damage, vision problems, loss of coordination of movement (ataxia), nerve pain, lack of sensitivity in the legs (peripheral neuropathy), arrhythmia, damage to the memory (in particular in the short-term and working memory), anxiety, depression with the danger of suicide, change of personality with loss of emotion and urge control, and permanent irritation. These are slow, long-term effects that cause progressive loss of the will to live and the desire to maintain social relationships.

The same high stress resulted in the Mosel region of Germany from eight treatments of the vineyards per year with organic phosphorus pesticides sprayed from airplanes.

Progressive neurodegeneration grows worse for many years after the end of exposure to organic phosphorus pesticides, so that the personality continues to deteriorate. The PET topography of persons affected showed impairment in particular in the prefrontal lobe, which is important for weighing up advantages and disadvantages and for taking decisions; and in the gyrus frontalis inferior, which is important overall for the personality and moral behaviour, as well as for motivation coordination, short-term memory and problem-solving strategies. The visual cortex was also damaged (gyrus orbitalis). The relevant personality changes usually led to withdrawal and social isolation and to suicidal tendencies[79, 80].

The toxic group of molecules of organic phosphates blocks degradation of acetylcholine, causing this neurotransmitter to build up in the brain. Thus acetylcholine binds to stimulating muscarinic receptors, from where the glutamate receptors are stimulated, and this leads to general overexcitation in the central nervous system. Glutamic acid activates the N-methyl-D-aspartate receptor (NMDA), which is important for learning. However, this causes pathological inflammation.

The muscarinic receptors occur in the frontal lobes, the hippocampus (important for memory capacity) and the basal ganglia. Excessive activation of these receptors further promotes the inflammatory processes. Permanent overstimulation of the NMDA receptor is deemed a primary cause of neurodegeneration through pesticides that destroys the mitochondria of all cells, lipid peroxidation of the cell membranes and myelin sheaths, and nerve cells by apoptosis.

Further neurotoxic harmful substances are used in daily life and at the workplace, as well as in family gardens: pesticides of the semi-synchronistic pyrethroid, type which are sold in any drug store and which providers recommend for use against vermin in the household and garden. They have a high neurotoxic potential.

Other neurotoxic heavy metals are found in batteries, accumulators, paints, jewellery, ceramic glazings, electronic devices and construction materials; these include cadmium, lead, thallium, nickel and chrome. They are often not disposed of as stipulated.

Other neurotoxic substances are found in flame retardants, such as polybromated diphenyl ether (PBDE) and tetrabrombisphenol A (TBBA). These substances are found in upholstery, electronic devices, carpets and cuddly toys for children. From there they slowly and continually enter the human organism and accumulate in the lipid-containing myelin sheaths of the brain. Since 1972, the content of toxic bromated flame retardants in breast milk has doubled every five years.

Wood-protection agents and neurodegenerative diseases

Pentachlorophenol (PCP) has been prohibited since 1989, because it causes cancer and neurodegenerative diseases. In many old buildings, however, it is still present and emitting toxic vapours. Since the 1970s and 1980s, treatment of all prefabricated buildings containing PCP has been required. The neurotoxic effect of the newer replacement substances for PCP, among them dichlor-fluanid, has not been sufficiently investigated. Hazardous long-term effects are quite possible.

Neurotoxic medicines and neurodegeneration

Prescription of neuroleptics of the family of the phenothiazine and butyrophenone drugs in psychiatric clinics and practices is widespread. They cause the symptoms of

Parkinson's disease by blocking the post-synaptic dopamine receptors and thus inhibiting the dopamine effect of the substantia nigra. Reserpine, as an isolated medicine or in Rauwolfia preparations, lowers the blood pressure and has a calming effect. It inhibits the presynaptic release of dopamine and may therefore trigger Parkinson symptoms.

Legal and prohibited drugs and neurodegenerative diseases

Cannabis

The active substances of cannabis, including tetrahydrocannabinol (THC), activate a dedicated group of receptors, mostly in the cerebral cortex (CB 1 und CB 2). The nerve cells activated by this are connected to many others that, when affected by cannabis, release various neurotransmitters, such as acetylcholine, noradrenaline, dopamine, serotonin and glutamate.

As a *primary effect* of the drug, there is an increase in sensory impressions and sensations, changes in the perception of time, increases in feelings of well-being and self-esteem, relaxation and a reduction in the perception of pain.

The *secondary effects (withdrawal effects)* are: hallucinations, anxiety, laughing fits, vertigo, impaired perception, delusions, paranoia and fatigue.

The neurotoxic long-term effects of cannabis are: memory and concentration disorders, motivation deficits, loss of drive, fatigue and idleness, increased risk of schizophrenia, psychotic episodes, brain damage and brain shrinkage (especially in the nucleus amygdalae).

Amphetamines

Amphetamines stimulate the release of monoamine neurotransmitters, such as serotonin, noradrenaline and dopamine. At the same time, they inhibit monoamine oxidase (MAO-inhibition), so that breakdown of excess neurotransmitters is delayed, especially in the area of the brain stem ganglia and the limbic system, where memory contents are linked to emotions.

The *primary effects* of methamphetamine, paramethoxyamphetamine (PMA) and other (Ecstasy) drugs are: stimulation, improved physical performance, increased vigilance (awareness), reduced thirst and hunger, loss of inhibition, enhanced ego.

The *secondary effects (withdrawal effects)* are: sleeplessness, fear, depression, speech disorders, hallucinations, delusions, psychosis (schizophrenia), high blood pressure, high pulse rate. After large doses: cramps, respiratory arrest and kidney failure.

The *neurotoxic long-term effects* are: fatigue, sleeping disorders, emaciation, high blood pressure, paranoid hallucination, learning and memory disorders, a decline in intelligence, psychoses, dementia, degeneration of serotonin and dopamine-expressing nerves in the hippocampus and limbic system, increased risk of stroke and damage to the heart muscle (toxic myopathy).

LSD (lysergic acid diethylamide)

This drug has an activating effect on serotonin-(5-HT)-receptors in various brain areas, mostly in the brain stem, which are connected to the limbic system.

Primary effects of this drug are: hallucinations in colourful imaginary images, increased sensory perception, overstimulation.

The *secondary effects (withdrawal effects)* are: loss of control of the body and of thinking, impaired space-time perception, concentration and attention disorders, balance disorders, panic, delusions.

The *neurotoxic long-term effects* are: hallucinations and loss of a sense of reality. The potential for psychological addiction is mode- rate and that of physical addiction is low.

Heroin, morphine, other opiates

Opiates release endorphins.

Primary effect: euphoria (feelings of unnatural joy and excessive well-being), sedation (sleepiness), much reduced perception of pain, dullness, inhibition, enhanced ego, reduced perception (apathy towards others and oneself), reduced morality, respiratory arrest.

Secondary effects (withdrawal symptoms): lower blood pressure, slow pulse (bradycardia), fatigue, apathy, nausea, vertigo and considerable oversensitivity to pain in the body and limbs.

Neurotoxic long-term effect: Depression, mood swings, sleep disorder, mood lability, lack of drive, visual hallucinations, personality change

Cocaine

Primary effect: An unnatural elation, increased self-confidence and mental euphoria, increased mental activity for a brief duration (a little over an hour). Lack of criticism in decisions and towards oneself, reduced perception of responsibility, reduced perception of guilt, accelerated breathing, tachycardia.

Secondary effects (withdrawal symptoms): Fear, hallucinations, panic, paranoia, nausea, depression, enormous addiction potential, procurement crime.

Neurotoxic long-term effect: Apathy, lack of orientation, reduced judgement, fatigue, drowsiness, weak focus, premature aging of the entire organism, reduced life expectancy, strongly premature aging of the brain (brain shrinking at twice the normal speed (atrophy), particularly of the prefrontal cortex and the temporal lobe, loss of memory and judgement, dementia.

Nicotine

Nicotine also stimulates the acetylcholine receptors in the vegetative centres of the brain stem and the medulla oblongata, where the centres for blood pressure, respiration and the heart are situated. The ganglia of the sympathicus and parasympathicus (vagus) are stimulated at a lower dose and inhibited at a higher dose, until there is a receptor blockage. In the stimulation phase, neurotransmitters are released in various areas of the brain, among them dopamine, adrenaline, noradrenaline, acetylcholine, serotonin and β-endorphin. The blocking of these receptors is reflected in the secondary effect. High persistent doses of nicotine (chain smokers) will cause only the secondary and toxic symptoms.

Primary effect: cognitive performance, memory, attention, inhibition of fear, stress, pain, positive feelings.

Secondary effects (withdrawal symptoms): fast pulse, high blood pressure, nervousness, restlessness, impatience, sleeping disorder, irritability, inability to concentrate, reduced performance, reduced attention, sensitivity to pain, negative emotions.

Neurotoxic long-term effect: very strong physical and psychological addiction, discomfort, depression, toxic effects of heavy metals in cigarette smoke.

Other toxic effects: arteriosclerosis, cerebral sclerosis, heart attack, stroke, strongly increased cancer risk (benzo[a]pyrene), emphysema of the lung.

Nicotine during pregnancy is neurotoxic for the unborn child. Smoking during pregnancy increases the risk of noticeable behavioural problems in later life that is 1.9 times as large; the risk is particularly high for ADHS syndrome (Attention Deficit Hyperactivity Syndrome). Exposure of the child to passive smoke after birth causes a 1.3 times increase in the risk of later behavioural disorders for the child. Smoking during pregnancy and passive smoke exposure after birth double this risk for the child.

Alcohol

Alcohol is fat-soluble and therefore penetrates the blood-brain barrier, so that the toxic effect on the nerve cells (neurons), glial cells and myelin sheaths is the main issue. Alcohol harms the blood-brain barrier directly and so severely that the brain becomes more susceptible to other toxins.

Primary effect: disinhibition, talkativeness, euphoric mood, reduced ability to think and make judgements, incapacity to control urges, sleepiness or aggressive behaviour, lack of emotional detachment, paralysis, speech and balance problems, blurred perception, loss of judgement ability, loss of consciousness leading to coma.

Secondary effects (withdrawal symptoms): vertigo, vomiting, headache, slower reactions, sleeping, balance and coordination problems, tremor, delirium tremens, paralysis, inability to think clearly, dulled thought processes, depression, irritability.

Neurotoxic long-term effect: loss of mental capacity, reduced ability to make judgements, ethylic dementia, personality changes, polyneuropathy with vitamin B1 and zinc deficit (sensory impairment, pain), disrupted relationships, paranoia (paranoid ideas, paranoia persecutoria), destruction of personality, social decline.

Other toxic effects: Other toxic effects: severe liver damage, cirrhosis of the liver, pancreatitis and pancreatic cancer, increased risk of cardiovascular diseases, heart attack and stroke, chronic atrophic gastritis (stomach inflammation) with vitamin B12-deficit, anaemia and degeneration of the sensitive pathways of the spinal cord.

Alcohol consumption during pregnancy Analysis of several studies showed significant interrelations between the moderate alcohol consumption of the mother and development of ADHS syndrome in the child, starting with one glass of wine per week[81]. Thus even very low levels of alcohol during pregnancy will cause foetal alcohol syndrome (FAS), with significant mental disability in the child.

Caffeine

The neurons (brain cells) have receptors for adenosine. When overstimulated and when their functions are overloaded, they produce adenosine, which binds to their receptors. This reduces the reception of stimuli by the neurites, which is reflected in mental fatigue, slower thinking and inability to concentrate.

Caffeine binds to the adenosine receptors of the neurons of the brain and displaces adenosine. This sabotages the protective natural blockage that normally allows the brain cells to recover and restores the ability to think and remain vigilant (wakefulness) for 1–2 hours.

Constantly repeated caffeine consumption in the form of coffee or 'energy drinks' contributes to chronic fatigue and degenerative changes in the neurons. Caffeine activates the stress hormone axis, so that adrenaline and cortisol are produced to a greater extent. This causes increased formation of cytokines and susceptibility to inflammation, also in the central nervous system.

Primary effect: restoration of vigilance (wakefulness) and clear thinking, brightening of mood, fast pulse, rise in blood pressure.

Secondary effects (withdrawal symptoms): increased fatigue, slower mental processes, sleepiness during the day, sleeping disorders at night, irritability, restlessness, insomnia, headache, overacidification of the stomach, impaired stomach and intestinal peristalsis. Reduced mental performance as a secondary effect after even just a single cup of coffee can be documented in psychological performance tests for up to one week after consumption.

Neurotoxic long-term effects: nervous mental exhaustion, headache and migraines. Bypassing the natural protective effect of the neurons leads to the expectation that caffeine might be a contributory cause for neuro degenerative diseases. Scientific examination of this is still inadequate.

Other toxic long-term effects of regular coffee consumption: migraine headaches, high blood pressure, increased risk of cardiovascular diseases, heart attack, stroke, heartburn from reflux, stomach and duodenal ulcers, stomach cancer, increased risk of many cancer types from the carcinogenic contents of coffee (not from caffeine).

Regarding the phenomenon of primary and secondary effects and the danger of polypragmasia from medication

Primary effects are the first reaction to a medicine or a drug. After the relevant duration, which is specific to each drug, there will be a counter-regulation on the part of the organism that causes a secondary effect or reaction which is usually not desired. This phenomenon is generally not sufficiently taken into consideration when prescribing medicines, so that secondary effects are often viewed as a new symptom and further medicines are prescribed for them. The undesired side effects of medicines are typically secondary effects. When more than two drugs or medicines are taken, the interactions between the medicines can no longer be traced. Therefore the body's reaction cannot be predicted.

Undesired neurotoxic side effects of prescribed medicines are common. They are very well recorded and described in medicine compendiums and files, as well as in packaging leaflets. To prevent neurodegenerative diseases, both the prescribing doctor and the patient must consider the undesired neurotoxic effects.

The combined effect of harmful neurotoxic substances

The effects of stresses from heavy metals, formaldehyde, dioxins, pesticides, solvents, drugs (including alcohol, nicotine and caffeine) accumulate so that compliance with the limits for individual substances when combined with others should be at a much lower level than what is today acceptable for the individual substance alone.

Vitamins, trace elements and neurodegenerative disease

Vitamins A, C, E act as antioxidants in the metabolism. Vitamins A, D, E and K are fat-soluble. In the case of a massive overdose for an extended period of time, they may have a neurotoxic effect. A lack of vitamin B_6 and zinc prevents neurotransmitters from forming sufficiently. A chronic pesticide stress will cause vitamin B_6 and zinc deficiencies.

A low blood level of the reduced form of folic acid (5 methyltetrahydrofolic acid) is associated with depression[82]. Where there is a vitamin-C deficiency, folic acid can only be converted into its reduced form (5-MTHF) in insufficient amounts. This reduced form (5-MTHF) is necessary, however, to convert homocysteine into methionine in combination with vitamin B12 in order to then form S-Adenosyl methionine. This is necessary for the formation of monoamine neurotransmitters. Additionally, reduced folic acid (5-MTHF) is needed for synthesis of adrenaline from noradrenaline in the adrenal gland.

A deficiency of folic acid causes the metabolism of the nervous system to become oversensitive to oxidative stress. This is indicated by an increased homocysteine level in the blood, which is due to a deficit of natural antioxidants, vitamin C, glutathione and NADH (nicotinamide adenine dinucleotide hydrogen). Accordingly, infusions with glutathione, vitamin C, folic acid and vitamin B_{12} have proven effective in treating persons with depression. A high homocysteine level, combined with a low concentration of B-vitamins (folic acid, vitamin B_{12}, vitamin B_6) is considered to be a risk factor for Alzheimer's disease and vascular dementia (dementia due to arteriosclerosis and vascular occlusion)[83]. Thus a high homocysteine level is regarded as a prognostic marker for the presence of a high risk of developing dementia. In 65-year-old patients, it can often be found together with a deficit in folic acid as well as in vitamins B_6 and B_{12}. This constellation is regarded as a preliminary stage of Alzheimer's disease. At the same time, it is an expression of oxidative stress from poor nutrition, an unnatural lifestyle, lack of sleep, chronic inflammation as in diabetes, then rheumatic inflammations, autoimmune inflammations and detrimental environmental influences (e.g. exposure of toxins and radiation), depression and Alzheimer's disease.

Vitamin D deficit is common today. Only the UVB-spectrum of sunlight, falling directly on the skin, will enable its production in its active form in a sufficient amount. The intestines resorb it only to a small degree. At low altitudes (below 1,200 metres above sea level), sunlight only contains the full UVB spectrum during the summer months, since it is absorbed in the vapour layers when the sunlight is at a low angle of incidence to the surface of the earth. Sun blockers, including those with a very low protection factor, cut out precisely that spectrum of the sunlight. Therefore more frequent exposure to the sun with the head covered but without sun blocker, for a duration of 20 minutes for each side of the body in the summer months, is particularly important for storing the greatest possible amount of vitamin D in the liver as a stock for the winter months.

Vitamin-D substitution reduces the depots of β-amyloid in the inter-cellular tissue of the brain and thus protects against Alzheimer's disease[84]. An increasing number of epidemiological studies indicates that vitamin-D deficiency is associated with a large number of different neuropsychiatric and neurodegenerative diseases[85], including multiple sclerosis[86, 87].

The diversity of causes of neurodegenerative diseases

We have seen that there are many diverse causes for neurodegenerative diseases. However, only a few rare cases have genetic causes. In most – and particularly in the most common neurodegenerative diseases, such as multiple sclerosis, Parkinson's disease, Alzheimer's disease and amyotrophic lateral sclerosis – experts cannot reach agreement, since these diseases always have multiple causes and researchers usually deal with them one at a time. More and more scientific evidence for the relevance for neurodegenerative diseases of widespread poor nutrition (i.e. industrially synthesised food high in sugar, white flour, animal fats and proteins, but low in polyunsaturated fatty acids and vegetarian fresh food, with alcohol, coffee and other stimulants and toxins) has been collected in recent years. Its relevance is surely still considerably underestimated, however. The causative relevance of many neurotoxins has been thoroughly researched, while the causative relevance of radiation stress will probably become evident in the next few years. The relevance of an orderly lifestyle adjusted to the biological requirements of human life, as well as orderly sleep, is also still greatly underestimated, even though the effect of stress, harassment and bullying and other mental traumas as causative factors for neurodegenerative diseases has already been researched in a neuropsychiatric context.

Assuming a multifactorial cause of such severe diseases, the only possible way to prevent and – where still possible – heal them is to include all causative factors that can be influenced within the treatment plan. This book is based on this insight and on many decades of experience in the very successful prevention and treatment of neurodegenerative diseases, Alzheimer's and vascular dementia, multiple sclerosis and efficient prevention of other neurodegenerative diseases.

The various types of neurodegenerative diseases

All known neurodegenerative diseases are listed here systematically to provide an overview. Most of these conditions are rare congenital diseases. This book will focus only on Alzheimer's disease, vascular dementia and Lewy body dementia, in which genetics plays no role or only a minor one. However, the therapeutic measures described in this book can influence the progress and condition of patients positively even in genetically caused neurodegenerative diseases. The prevention and treatment of multiple sclerosis, Parkinson's disease, amyotrophic lateral sclerosis and Guillain-Barré syndrome are discussed in Bircher-Benner manual no. 1: 'Multiple sclerosis, Parkinson's disease and other neurodegenerative diseases'.

Systematic overview of neurodegenerative diseases

Diseases resulting from destructive degenerative proteins: (TAU proteins:
– Alzheimer's disease
– Progressive supranuclear palsy (PSP)
– Corticobasal degeneration(CBD)
– Argyrophilic grain disease (AGD)
– Frontotemporal dementia, Parkinsonism of the chromosome 17 (FTDP17)
– Pick's disease

Synucleinopathies:
– Parkinson's disease (PD)
– Lewy body dementia (LBD)
– Multiple system atrophy (MSA)

TDP-34 Proteinopathies:
– Frontotemporal lobe degeneration with TDP 34

FUS pathies:
– Frontotemporal lobe degeneration with FUS (FTDL-FUS)
– Neuronal intermediate filament inclusion disease (NIFID)
– Basophilic inclusion body disease (BIBD)

Trinucleotide diseases:
– Huntington's disease (HD)
– Spinal and bulbar muscular atrophy, Kennedy type (SBMA)
– Friedreich's ataxia (FA)
– Spinocerebellar ataxia (SCA)
– Dentatorubro-pallidoluysian atrophy (DRPLA)

Prion diseases:
– Creutzfeldt-Jakob disease
– Gerstmann-Sträussler-Scheinker syndrome
– Fatal familial insomnia
– Kuru

Diseases of the motor neurons:
– Amyotrophic lateral sclerosis (ALS)
– Primary lateral sclerosis
– Spinal muscular atrophy (SMA)

Neuroaxonal dystrophies:
– Infantile neuroaxonal dystrophy Seitelberger
– Neurodegeneration with brain iron accumulation (NBIA)

Unclassifiable neurodegenerative diseases:
- Frontotemporal lobe degeneration with ubiquitin proteasome system (FTLD-UPS)
- Familiar encephalopathy with neuroserpin inclusions
- CANVAS (Cerebellar ataxia neuropathy, vestibular areflexia syndrome)

Multiple sclerosis

Parkinson's disease

Amyotrophic lateral sclerosis

Guillain-Barré syndrome

Peripheral neuropathies

Dementia

Dementia diseases produce unspeakable suffering. Dementia commences with a gradual loss of short-term memory. Clarity of thought, speech and motor skills decline as a result. Ultimately long-term memory suffers too, leading to a loss of early memories and the skills acquired in life. Patients suffer from immense fears, experience loss and isolation, and develop a deep distrust towards people and their environment. Orientation in time and space dissipates until even the most familiar persons are no longer recognised. Consciousness is not affected. The patients are not shielded against fully perceiving the tragic situation.

Diagnosis of dementia

For diagnosis, the memory loss must be accompanied by at least one of the following disorders: speech disorder (aphasia), a loss of the ability to perform certain movements correctly (apraxia), a loss of the ability to recognise certain objects (agnosia) or a loss of the ability to plan and organise actions correctly and to comply with a certain sequence (dysexecutive syndrome).

Forms of dementia

Neuropsychiatry distinguishes many forms of dementia based on cause. The most frequent forms are not inherited, but rather are caused by degenerative diseases.

Alzheimer's dementia is by far the most frequent form (approx. 60%). The rare forms are included in the overview:

Degenerative forms of dementia:
– Morbus Alzheimer
– Frontotemporal dementia
– Lewy body dementia

Vascular dementia (VAD)
This results from changes to the vessels in the brain due to various causes:

Multi-infarct syndrome:
This results from one or several vascular occlusions from arteriosclerosis or blood clots that reach the brain vessels (embolisms).

Strategic lesions:
These result from vascular occlusions at a small scope that occur in critical locations that interfere with the mental abilities.

Microangiopathic lesions:
These result from progressive arteriosclerosis in small brain vessels.

Micro-vascular changes:
These result when there is a widespread loss of capillary vessels in the brain and damage to the blood-brain barrier.

Forms of genetically inherited vascular dementia:
CADASIL disease, HERNS syndrome, genetic English, Dutch or Icelandic forms of dementia with deposition of degenerative proteins (amyloidosis).

Forms of dementia as a consequence of other general diseases
- dementia in the late stage of Parkinson's disease
- dementia from inflammation of the brain in AIDS (HIV)
- dementia from epilepsy
- dementia from inherited hepatolenticular degeneration (Morbus Wilson)
- dementia from calcium deposits at an excessive and persistent calcium level (hypercalcemia)
- dementia from sustained underactivity of the thyroid gland (hypothyreosis)
- dementia from poisoning (intoxication)
- dementia in the late stage of multiple sclerosis
- dementia in Panarteritis nodosa (auto-allergic arterial inflammation)
- dementia in the late stage of systemic Lupus erythematosus
- dementia from niacin or vitamin B_{12} deficit
- dementia from disturbances of the lipid metabolism
- dementia from Pick's disease
- dementia from Creutzfeldt-Jakob's disease
- dementia in the late stage of genetic Huntington's Chorea

Dementia becomes more and more frequent

Since 1997, it has become clear that, in the USA and for the first time, dementia among older people is growing more and more frequent. Additionally, about every other older person is not diagnosed[88]. According to the 2015 global Alzheimer's report, 46.8 million people in the world supposedly suffer from dementia. That number is expected to rise to 74.1 million by 2030[89].
According to a study conducted in Berlin, 1.2 % of those aged 60–70, 2.7 % of those aged 70–74, 6 % of those aged 75–79, 13.3 % of those aged 80–83, 23.9 % of those aged 85–89 and 34.6 % of those older than 90 suffered from dementia. In Germany alone, three million people are expected to suffer from dementia by 2050[90]. Congenital forms are rare. The strong and continuous increase of dementia refers to the forms of dementia that result from neuro- and other degenerative diseases.

Officially accepted risk factors of dementia

Symptomatic treatments and interventions, in particular in cardiology and cardiac surgery, have led to slightly increased lifespans in industrialised countries[91]. That age is the greatest risk factor for dementia is no longer accepted as a matter of course by some authorities and scientists. It is often noted that industrial countries show a correlation between old age and dementia. However, this does not lead to the conclusion that age is the most important cause of dementia. A counter-argument often cites the elderly Japanese on Okinawa island, in which no causality of old age and dementia can be established.

On the other hand, it is accepted that women are affected more often due to their longer life expectancy.

Sustained depression will cause the hippocampus to atrophy and can lead to dementia more often. However, depression can also be an early symptom of the onset of dementia and significantly precedes memory loss. In particular those people who suffer from dementia early are often depressed. The impairment of the mental abilities in psychoses and depression is often difficult to distinguish from dementia, creating a risk of misdiagnosis. Other accepted risk factors are those that also apply to cardiovascular diseases, such as metabolic syndrome with obesity, diabetes, disorders of the fat metabolism, lack of movement, smoking, but also renal insufficiency and an increased homocysteine level in the blood as a signifier of oxidative stress. Fighting these risk factors effectively reduces the risk of suffering from dementia clearly[92, 93, 94, 95, 96, 97]. A long-term study over four years of 4425 Japanese people aged 65 and older showed that the risk of developing dementia was increased by 1.85 times if 13 or more teeth were missing and not replaced[98]. People who are unable to chew well will select their food differently. Pre-digestion in the mouth by means of saliva is also strongly impaired.

The symptoms of dementia

The gradual loss of short-term memory is a leading symptom of dementia. In particular those people who maintained a lot of social contact in their lives will often be able to cover this up for a long time in superficial contact. Later, a pervasive change of character will occur. Interests decline, and patients no longer enjoy what they used to. They become irritable and subdued, and feel overburdened by everyday things that before were not burdensome. Burdened by distrust towards themselves and others, they slowly slip into loneliness and total isolation. Soon relatives and friends will notice this change of character and its tragic effects. They will notice that actions or statements are repeated without sense or that noticeable nonsensical actions are performed. Arithmetic becomes impossible, words are hard to find and orientation in everyday life and in space becomes more and more difficult, so that even the smallest changes to their usual environment, such as a construction site, will render patients unable to find their way home. Distrust and fear become tormenting, to which soon are added immense fatigue and apathy. In the late stage, patients will slip into total isolation since they cannot even recognise their closest relatives anymore. They become extremely agitated or apathetic, bedridden and incontinent. Dementia as such does not cause death, but it facilitates diseases that ultimately kill the patients.

Usually the patients also suffer from movement disorders, such as Parkinson's shaking palsy. Their bodies gradually become stiff. They start to walk with small and dragging steps, with their legs far apart. Their postural reflexes are impaired and they are at risk of falling.

Patients with dementia lose initiative. They easily feel ordered around because they can no longer understand their relatives' desire to help in the context of the current situation. They neglect their former hobbies and personal hygiene, and no longer tidy up at home. Then they are no longer able to eat sufficiently, they lose their appetite, and finally they forget to chew and swallow food. This causes them to grow emaciated (marasmus), weakens them and renders them susceptible to infections and other internal diseases.

Their day/night rhythm is completely impaired, which can be very difficult for nurses.

The patients also often suffer from eating disorders. Two-thirds of them eat inedible things, become highly agitated, and are unstable and aggressive. Every other patient suffers from massive sleeping disorders, depression, fear and delusions. Every forth patient with dementia suffers from massive disinhibition and hallucinations, and every seventh of an unnaturally from jubilant mood (euphoria)[99].

Psychotic symptoms such as hallucinations and delusions can occur in any form of dementia, but are particularly found in

Parkinson's syndrome and Lewy body dementia. Visual hallucinations are quite typical. Patients see persons who are not present, in twilight conditions, and will fearfully talk to them, even though they may realise in the beginning that they are not actually there. Later they will see patterns on walls – animals or mythological creatures or dust mites. They will panic as they experience scenic hallucinations, such as kidnapping, and even delirium. It is easily understandable that in such conditions of delusion they may become highly aggressive towards their families and the people who are trying to help them.

Those suffering from the onset of dementia lose their standing in society. This leads to great mental pain, isolation and fear. They are quickly labelled as 'written-off, worthless and in need of help'. Some thoughtless people call them 'a strain on society'[100, 101].

Diagnosis of dementia

Diagnosis is not simple. Dementia must be distinguished from temporary impairment of the ability to remember and think. Information provided by the patients and their family members is particularly important. The information of the patient on increasing loss of memory is considered a highly reliable indication for early recognition of the onset of dementia[102]. Lab examinations help determine the blood levels of homocysteine, folic acid, vitamin B_{12} and fasting blood glucose, renal and hepatic values, electrolytes and thyroid hormones. An electroencephalogram (EEG) and magnetic resonance imaging (MR) are needed to determine the cause. Simple psychometric tests can be conducted to review the scope of memory impairment (MMSE test, clock test, DEM test).

To permit initiation of the right treatment, dementia must be distinguished from syphilis, the consequences of depression, deprivation in the nursing home, delirium, psychoses, simple mutism, avoidance and aphasia (loss of speech).

Diagnostic options have greatly improved recently. It is now possible to recognise Alzheimer's disease at an early stage with only mild cognitive impairment (MCI-stage). Neuroradiologically even a slight reduction (atrophy) of the middle temporal lobe or hippocampus can now be recognised. Increase of the τ- and β-amyloids in the cerebral fluid can be measured. Positron emission tomography (PET) can be used to recognise reduced glucose uptake in degenerating brain areas. Alzheimer's disease can thus be distinguished from Pick's disease (frontotemporal dementia) or chronic depression, for example. A PET-CT can visually reveal amyloid deposits in the brain. With a clinical score that can be used in any medical practice, the onset of Alzheimer's disease can be recognised early (80 % reliability) without any technical tools[103]. PET-CT with L-dopa and Iodine-123-IBZM-scintigraphy can recognise forms of dementia in Parkinson's disease, multiple system atrophy (MSA), essential tremor or progressive supranuclear palsy early on and distinguish them from each other.

Notes on care and nursing for persons suffering from dementia

The risk of loss of mental skills and the fear of dependence constitute an enormous threat, in addition to a significant loss of respect and support in society. It is easily understandable that people will try to conceal the newly occurring damage by any means. Family members recognising the change must never judge. They must first try to lovingly encourage the affected person to undergo careful diagnosis, and then support them throughout the process. This is often not possible immediately and may take time. Experience has shown that one must also caution against hasty judgements made on the basis of imaging procedures, even PET-CT.

It has often paid off to use the time preceding complete diagnosis to investigate all possible causes and to initiate intense dietary therapy, detoxing and antioxidative infusion treatment. In our experience, such measures have caused numerous premature diagnoses to dissipate, with subsequent magnetic resonance imaging again showing normal results. However, this investigation and exclusion of possible causes and treatment must commence immediately. No time must be lost, since the damage to the brain will have started long before the first symptoms appeared.

When clearly diagnosed that degenerative dementia is already present, it has proven valuable to continue to exercise caution and to inform the patients only to the extent that they wish. It is best for them to focus on therapeutic means and on remaining skills. Patients understandably avoid situations in which they are conflicted with their new weaknesses, in order to avoid threatening situations, fear and insults. Such attempts at self-protection must not be hampered.

Depending on the stage of the disease, it is often difficult to ascertain which information the patient is able to absorb. The best time to talk to patients about their impairment is when they themselves ask about the causes of their problems.

Giving them the diagnosis 'Alzheimer's disease' can cause people to fall into deep resignation. It is better to generally speak of a disease that may affect learning and orientation and that will now be fought with all means. This is all the more important since diagnosis of Alzheimer's disease during life always remains uncertain. If patients endanger themselves by refusing urgently needed help, it may be necessary to talk to them about their impairments even though they do not wish to listen. In that case, it is important to try to prevail in the calmest and most relaxed manner possible. Never let yourself slip into an aggressive or depreciating attitude. Rather, always take a diplomatic approach that will enable patients to experience themselves as competent and able to make decisions in spite of their condition. Perceiving one's own deficits will often lead to resignation. An appraising and supporting attitude in family members and nurses can then be decisive.

It is important to remember that dementia not only leads to memory disorders but also to changes in how patients think, feel and behave. Therefore perception of family members gradually changes. In light of this it is not easy, though it is very important, to accept the patients in spite of all of these changes, and to show as much understanding and tolerance as possible for their behaviour.

The abilities of persons suffering from dementia may fluctuate greatly over the course of a given day. Moments of weakness may be mistaken for unwillingness. When strangers are present, patients with dementia often try as hard as they can to make a good impression to avoid the pain of disappointment and contempt. This is possible only for a very limited time, after which they will give up in exhaustion.

Time pressure, stress and a hectic pace will very quickly drive persons with dementia into mental blocks and emotional reactions that they are no longer able to control, such as anger, fury, irritation and uncontrollable crying.

Persons with dementia often suffer from melancholia and depression, and they lose all courage. They often say 'I don't care about anything', or 'It's all over'. Sometimes they talk of suicide. They often lose drive and appetite, and they become insomniac. Their emotions immediately spread to their family members and nurses. It is very important to recognise at once that the emotions we feel are initially those of the patient, and not our own. Only this will enable us not to take patients' behaviour personally and interpret it as being ungrateful. This is done best by listening and trying to inspire patients to activities they used to like and can still do well. Music therapy and art therapy (painting therapy) may be a great help here, since these forms of therapy do not have any evaluations or ideas of performing. These therapies are meant to give patients a means of expression and to participate in a shared activity.

People have generally forgotten how to sing. Their apartments are now usually filled by restless, disharmonious sounds or squeaky pop voices from electronic devices. Persons with dementia are made restless and fearful by this. It can be a great help to sing songs together that the patients know from their childhood.

Patients with dementia are often driven by restlessness, so that they must walk around their apartments or will run away from home without any clear destination. Maybe they grew bored or they are driven by fear or feel that they are in the wrong location. The reasons for running away are often unknown to the patient. Nothing should be changed inside the home if possible, so that patients feel at home and know their way around it. Patients who cannot find their way home would benefit from small transmitters that can locate patients at any time by means of a GPS-localization system. The same localization device can be used by patients to inform those persons looking for a lost patient.

Even with the best of intentions, do not try to train patients with memory exercises, calculations or abstract mental demands. Only those things which patients are able to accomplish through their own motivation and without time pressure can have a positive effect on them. In particular, talk to them about the skills they still consider themselves competent in.

It can be helpful to speak about early childhood memories to promote speech skills. The farther the disease has progressed, the more the patients will be reliving their earlier memories. It is good to meet them there. Walks in nature, in particular in the forest, speak to all sensory perceptions and will improve mood. It is good to talk about things you see together. This is much better than talking about abstract things that are difficult for the patients. Lots of movement and hiking are very important for maintaining and regenerating mental skills. It will also reduce fears and internal tensions.

It is very important to confront the patients with their deficits as little as possible and to correct their perception as little as possible. If they state any wrong perceptions, meet them there and show an understanding for what they see. When behaviour is corrected as inappropriate, patients with dementia are often particularly vulnerable, stubborn and irritable since they are confronted with loss of skill. They have trouble coping with this. Often it is better to tolerate anything diplomatically, unless it is dangerous. If the patient wears soiled clothes, it is better not to say this directly, but to choose beautiful, clean clothing for them and be visibly happy when they put it on.

The deepest needs are understanding, recognition, estimation and safety.

It is valuable to keep this in mind at all times. There is no simple and effective solution for some situations. In order to find solutions, it is important to learn to understand how the patient experiences and views the world. It may be worthwhile to participate in a group for family members of patients with dementia.

Most TV shows are recorded with a uselessly rapid image sequence. Even without dementia, most of them are only understood intuitively, since our awareness cannot follow what is shown in such a short period of time. The rapid image sequence bypasses conscious thought and may have severe consequences. This is all the more difficult for those suffering from dementia. Even in the early stages of dementia, patients will be at the mercy of the televised content even more than they used to be. In dementia of medium severity, what is shown can often no longer be distinguished from reality, so that existing fears are reawakened and enhanced, and new fears may occur.

From the early stages of dementia, it is very important that family members help structure the day so that joyful stimulation and restful breaks alternate. Persons at the onset of dementia often wonder about the meaning of their lives. Sometimes they are able to recognise that it feels good to hand over responsibilities that they themselves do not need to bear under all circumstances. Sometimes they can be encouraged to discover how pleasant it can be to help others who truly need it. It is also possible that they must be protected from freeloaders who claim that they need help.

Legal questions will arise in connection with driving initially.

When order therapy for Alzheimer's disease can be performed well and commences at an early stage, it is expected that the progress of dementia will soon slow considerably. The degenerative process can often be stalled, and skills can be regained. This makes it possible to turn towards positive things, and opens up a more acceptable future.

Nursing aids and risk reduction
Various risks exist in the household because of dementia. An automatic deactivator can be built into an electrical cooker. There are irons that turn off automatically when they are not moved for a certain short period of time. There are alarm mats that can be placed at the foot of the bed and the near the front door which will signal whenever the patient steps on them. Infrared motion detectors can be installed for similar purposes to help the patients. When getting up becomes difficult, a standing stool or rising device with an electrical motor may be sensible. There are protectors that reduce the risk of a femoral neck fracture in a fall by 80 %. An electrical nursing bed will be sensible at a later stage.

Legal issues
In the early stage of dementia, even the most important decisions can still be made by the patient. A notarised power of attorney can be used to issue a living will that determines what medical treatment is desired and under which circumstances. Additionally, patients can choose a person they trust who will take care of them if their condition deteriorates. If the patient is no longer able to do this or if this is not done, an official legal guardian should be appointed. It will be impossible to tell in advance if this person will actually be trustworthy. If the patient fears incapacitation by this step, it may help if a family member does it for themselves at the same time. In fact, everyone should do this. No one can know if they might become dependent due to accident or illness some day and need a legal guardian. Should this happen to, say, a spouse, it is

not a matter of course that the authority will appoint the other spouse as legal guardian. The notary public must emphasize the preventive character of this power of attorney and specify the powers of the authorised person in detail. If dementia was diagnosed by a doctor, unconsidered purchases made by the patient may be reversed. If the purchases were already paid for and the store refuses to take them back, this must be taken to court and the incapacity to make decisions must be demonstrated.

Additionally, preventive registration for a good seniors' residence and nursing home is sensible while one is still able to make such choices on one's own, even though it can be hoped that this step will never need to be taken. In the medium stage of dementia, nursing at home is usually no longer possible, except if one is able to pay for nursing staff around the clock. If family members put too much of a strain on themselves by nursing at home, they run a risk of contracting a severe disease, such as cancer, as well.

If restraining measures are needed in nursing homes in cases of severe dementia, such as bed barriers, straps or strong sedatives, the law requires that the authorised person or legal guardian be informed. If these measures are needed for an extended period of time, the person who is authorised to ensure the patient's well-being must consent in advance. The doctor may also only change medicines with this consent, in accordance with the law.

Driving cars is no longer permitted after a diagnosis of dementia. Should the patient drive notwithstanding this injunction, the liability insurance may refuse to pay, or may reduce payments or raise claims against the caregiver. Should the patient be unwilling to stop driving, the caregiver should initiate official review of the patient's ability to drive, in order to protect both the patient and others on the road.

The attending physician may and must also do this in spite of doctor-patient confidentiality.

Insurances
When dementia is diagnosed, it must be reported to the affected person's liability insurance, since insurance companies will see this as an increase of risk. If the dementia is not reported, insurance protection will be null and void. Doctors and nurses should also always carry liability insurance.

Alzheimer's disease

About 60 % of the approx. 26 million patients with dementia suffer from Alzheimer's dementia[104].

Alois Alzheimer was a German psychiatrist and neuropathologist. On 25 November 1901, he was entrusted with the treatment of 51-year-old Auguste Deter, who had changed dramatically in just a year. She had become jealous, was unable to do simple tasks in her household, hid things, felt persecuted and obstinately insulted her neighbours[105]. Her mental confusion quickly increased until she died of sepsis on 9 April 1902. Alzheimer examined her brain, which showed a mass destruction of nerve cells (neutrons) and massive deposits in the inter-cellular substance. On 3 November 1906, Alzheimer presented the case at a meeting at the University of Tübingen as a newly discovered, rare and independent disease. This was scarcely given any attention. His publication in the general psychiatry journal titled 'Über eine eigentümliche Krankheit der Hirnrinde' ('On a strange disease of the cerebral cortex') was not widely noticed either[106].

Over the next five years, 11 further cases were described until psychiatrist Emil Kraepelin included the disease in his new text book of psychiatry in 1910, calling it Morbus Alzheimer.

Alzheimer's disease, like vascular dementia and Lewy body dementia, is a primary form of dementia in which brain tissue is directly destroyed without involving any other disease as an immediate cause. Most people are only affected at an older age: 2 % of those aged 65, 3 % of those aged 70, 6 % of those aged 75 and 20 % of those aged 85. Frequency declines again at even higher ages. The youngest patient with Alzheimer's disease developed it at the age of 27 and died at 33[107].

Today, 1.3 million people in Germany suffer from dementia. By 2050, 2.5 million patients are expected with 250,000 new occurrences of dementia every year, including 120,000 of the Alzheimer's type[108]. Around the world, the number of patients with Alzheimer's disease was estimated at 29 million in 2007. Based on population forecasts of the United Nations Organisation (UNO), 106 million persons with Alzheimer's disease are expected by 2050. This corresponds to one person out of 85[109].

Many years before the first symptoms occur, deposits (plaques) form in the ground substance of the connective tissue (glia) in the patients' brains. These are made up of defectively folded degenerative, short-chained protein molecules (beta-β-amyloid (Aβ) peptides). Additionally, there are twisted fibrils of phosphorylated TAU proteins thereby rendered insoluble. These form dense balls in the nerve cells (neurons) and destroy them entirely.

Causes of Alzheimer's disease

Even though many causative factors are known, scientists are in disagreement, since they usually work on only one of them at a time.

Genetics
Genetics plays a subordinate role. It is estimated that no more than 30 % of the patients with Alzheimer's disease have genetic factors that contribute to their condition. There are families where Alzheimer's disease occurs frequently and at a relatively young age. In some, a variation of the gene for APO-E has been found. Additionally, mutations of the genes for formation of presenilin 1 or 2 or an amyloid predecessor protein (APP, amyloid precursor protein) were found. People in which all three of these genes are present are at risk of developing Alzheimer's disease more often and earlier than others. In such cases, an abundance of β-amyloid is deposited in the intracellular substance of the hippocampus and the prefrontal cortex (association cortex), and soon thereafter the entire brain. The genetic mutation for presenilin 1 (PSEN 1) on chromosome 14 or presenilin 2 (PSEN 2) on chromosome 1 or APP on chromosome 21 alone is found in 5–10 % of each of the patients with Alzheimer's disease. In 1,700 Icelandic persons, on the other hand, a different mutation was discovered in the APP gene, which protected against Alzheimer's disease[110].

The connection between Alzheimer's disease and the ε4 allele of apolipoprotein E (Apo E), which participates in cholesterol transport, is not yet clear. People who have three 21 chromosomes (trisomy 21, Down's syndrome, Mongolism) develop Alzheimer's disease about three times more often than people without this trisomy. In addition, a mutation of the SORL1 gene supposedly leads to a higher risk of Alzheimer's disease[111].

In about 1,000 persons who had emigrated from the Basque region to Columbian Antioquia, those affected by Alzheimer's disease showed a point mutation in the exon 8 of the PSEN 1 gene that occurs only in this specific group of people[112].

Infection hypothesis
Since the β-amyloids show a strong antibiotic effect, it has been suspected that they are excreted against pathogens so that a chronic infection may be a partial cause of Alzheimer's disease. This is disputed, however[113].

TAU proteins and Alzheimer's disease
Tests on mice showed that introduction of TAU proteins leads to the formation of twisted fibrils as in humans with Alzheimer's disease. Therefore, it is suspected that high blood levels of TAU proteins facilitate the development of Alzheimer's disease[114].

Head trauma increases the risk of developing Alzheimer's disease[115].

Many Alzheimer's risks are the same as those for cardiovascular disease and arteriosclerosis.
Fat metabolism disorders with increased cholesterol levels, diabetes with insulin resistance and increased insulin levels considerably increase the risk of Alzheimer's disease, as do metabolic syndrome with obesity and high blood pressure[116, 117, 118, 119, 120, 121].

Aluminium deposits
Aluminium from foods, deodorants, dishware, medicines and contaminated drinking water enters the brain and damages the blood-brain barrier (aluminium angiopathy)[122]. Aluminium contamination leads to deposits of aluminium in the ground substance of the connective tissue of the brain and contributes to deposits of β-amyloid in the Alzheimer plaques[123]. A meta-analysis of 34 studies on aluminium contamination and Alzheimer's disease has shown that 68 % of the studies documented a direct connection between aluminium deposits and Alzheimer's dis-

ease[124]. The British Alzheimer's society has held the medically scientific opinion since 30 January 2009 that the studies compiled until 2008 documented a causative connection between aluminium and Alzheimer's disease[125]. In April 2013, the European Food Safety Authority (EFSA) passed the recommendation that food should not be in contact with aluminium foil, since daily use of aluminium foil for storage of food will cause much more aluminium to enter the body than is tolerable according to the EFSA[126].

What happens in the brain at Alzheimer's disease

Amyloids are degeneratively changed, short-chained protein molecules. In Alzheimer's disease, β-amyloids deposit in the intercellular substance of the soft connective tissue (macroglia). The β-amyloid develops from a precursor protein (amyloid-precursor protein, APP). This is also called a membrane protein, since it penetrates the cell membrane of the nerve cell (neuron), with the short part protruding into the cell and the long part out of the cell into the intercellular space (matrix). This is also called the type I transmembrane protein. The amino terminus is located outside and the carboxyl terminus inside the cell. This precursor protein (APP) is split by three enzymes (alpha β-secretase, beta secretase and gamma secretase). This splitting produces the β-amyloid.

The amyloid-precursor protein (APP) is split in two different ways:

The non-amyloidogenic way

α secretase splits the APP molecule within the amyloid share and thereby prevents release of β-amyloid. For this, the largest part of this APP molecule outside of the cell is released. Its significance is not yet known.

The amyloidogenic way

The APP molecule is first cut by β-secretase and only then by γ secretase, in the location where the molecule penetrates the cell membrane. This releases β-amyloid.

β-amyloids are created with different lengths, which is very important. The longer the protein chain of the β-amyloid molecule, the more likely will it precipitate in the ground substance of the glia (matrix) and form insoluble plaques. Mostly, the Alzheimer plaques contain β-amyloid 40, and to a lesser extent β-amyloid 42. The numbers 40 and 42 correspond to the number of amino acids of which the amyloid peptide is made.

Proteases are protein-splitting enzymes

α secretase is formed by the proteases ADAM 10, ADAM 17 and TACE, β-secretase by the enzyme BACE 1.
γ secretase is highly complex. It consists of a large molecule complex: Presenilin 1, presenilin 2, PEN-2, APH-1 and nicastrin. It is suspected that other proteins are involved in this enzyme as well.

Every nerve cell contains approx. 1500 mitochondria. They are considered the power plants of the cells, by breaking down glucose step by step and forming high-energy phosphates (ATP), which are needed as energy donors anywhere in the metabolism. This is also called chemical „cell respiration". The mitochondria are made up of fine, biologically highly active membranes that are stabilised by lipids (fats) with polyunsaturated fatty acids. These membranes react highly sensitively to oxidation.

In Alzheimer's disease, the mitochondria are damaged by oxidative stress and partially destroyed. A block at the complex IV of the respiration chain in the mitochondria leads to excessive formation of free radicals (R.O.S.), which further damage the mitochondria. The β-amyloids have an antioxidant effect. Therefore, it is not certain whether they may also be formed to protect against free radicals.

The cell interior of the neurons contains TAU proteins (named after the Greek letter τ „TAU". The Tau proteins are dissolved inside the cell in healthy persons. Oxidative stress causes these protein molecules to form additional phosphor connections (hyperphosphorylation), until they become insoluble due to a bend in the molecule and are precipitated into twisted fibrils. These pathological twisted neurofibrils destroy the nerve cells and kill them (cell death = apoptosis).

This cell destruction typically starts in the hippocampus and the prefrontal cortex, which are structures that are relevant for memory and ordering thought. However, it may affect all areas of the brain. In imaging procedures, the reduction of brain mass (atrophy of the brain) and extension of the CSF spaces (spaces where cerebrospinal fluid is flowing) may be documented.

The symptoms of Alzheimer's disease

Recognising the first warning signs of Alzheimer's dementia is important for starting treatment as early as possible.

The 'American National Institute for Aging' formulated seven early warning signs:

1. Repeating the same question over and over.
2. Repeating the question the patient is asked.
3. Repetitive telling of the same anecdote.
4. Everyday work becomes impossible, including: cooking, operating a TV or radio, remembering the rules of a card game, etc.
5. Handling money, money transfers, checking and paying invoices and similar no longer possible.
6. Objects are placed in unusual and illogical locations and cannot be found anymore. Family members are accused of having taken them.
7. Neglecting outer appearance and care without realising it.

Tests can reveal warning signs for Alzheimer's dementia as early as eight years before the disease becomes noticeable. In the beginning, memory deteriorates and it becomes difficult to understand new information. Comprehension of speech and the pursuit of personal goals are also rendered difficult early on.
The mood soon darkens and apathy sets in[127, 128, 129].

The stages of the disease

At present, three stages of Alzheimer's disease can be distinguished:

1. The pre-clinical stage. The early signs are visible in tests, but the disease is not yet visible.
2. The stage of mild cognitive impairment (MCI). In this stage, impairment of mental capacities becomes clearly evident for the patients and their families.
3. The stage of dementia.

These stages merge together so that they are often difficult to distinguish from each other[130, 131].

Diagnosis of Alzheimer's disease

Diagnosis is possible only in the MCI stage of mild cognitive impairment. The diagnosis key ICD-10 distinguishes between G.30.0 (at early onset) and G30.1 (at late onset). Anamnesis with the patient and talks with family members, supplemented by neuropsychological testing and examination of the cerebral fluid (spinal tap, cerebrospinal fluid examination), are all very important. The diagnosis is secured by the direct amyloid presentation in the brain by positron emission tomography (PET) and radioactive marking, e.g. by Florbetaben[132, 133]. There is no reliable blood test for diagnosing Alzheimer's disease at the moment. The spinal tap may provide indications. The cerebrospinal fluid (liquor cerebrospinalis) may show an increased share of β-amyloids, total TAU proteins and phosphorylated TAU protein and some amyloid precursor proteins that provide diagnostic indications, but without securing any diagnosis[134].

Not every memory loss in old age is equivalent to Alzheimer's disease

A certain forgetfulness in advanced age is normal. Older people may also be unable to remember things because of refusal or avoidance. Cognitive inhibition due to depression is frequent in the elderly. Persistent depression will also cause the hippocampus to reduce (atrophy), as in Alzheimer's disease. Many old persons in seniors' residences suffer from isolation (emotional deprivation, hospitalism and regression) and thereby are inhibited in their thinking and memory capacities.

Aphasia (loss of the ability to speak) and mutism (refusal to speak for psychological reasons) are not rare in old age. Small or larger strokes can lead to vascular dementia. Mental illness (psychoses) such as schizophrenia or manic-depressive psychoses (cyclothymia) can lead to dementia. Other severe neurological disorders (apallic syndrome, locked-in syndrome, akinetic mutism) or damage by a brain tumour or after a brain injury can also be mistaken for Alzheimer's disease.

The early and medium stages of Alzheimer's disease

While processes and emotional experiences saved in long-term memory may still be available, loss of fresh memory when learning and loss of the ability to remember things will usually lead to diagnosis[135]. The ability to speak will soon decline, recognisable by the delayed flow of speech and reduced vocabulary. Nevertheless, patients can still share their thoughts and ideas in a suitable manner[136, 137, 138].

Insecurity in fine motor skills when writing, drawing or dressing soon appear (apraxia)[139]. When the medium stage of the disease begins, some patients may still be able to handle their everyday lives. However, they will need help with more complicated activities[140].

The later stage of Alzheimer's disease

Patients can no longer perform well-known activities. They are unable to recognise everyday objects or persons who are close to them[141, 142].

Change of character by Alzheimer's disease

The progressing destruction of brain tissue will lead to a change of character that is hard to understand and bear for the patients and their families. People who used to be peaceful and gentle will slowly lose control of their emotions. Distrust, accusations, paranoia and outbursts of rage become increasingly frequent and cause suffering for the patient and family members alike. It is harder and harder for them to recognise themselves (self-reflection). Behavioural patterns are uncontrolled and automated. This soon tries the patience of family members, even if they have the best intentions, and nursing at home will no longer be a viable option.

Physical deterioration of patients with Alzheimer's disease

In the third stage, the muscles deteriorate continually, which additionally leads to speech problems, and to urinary and faecal incontinence. Tragically patients lose their mobility. Small tentative steps are typical. They become bedridden. The simplest activities require help, and the need for nursing increases. The patients will soon die of infection, pneumonia or heart attack.

Life expectancy at Alzheimer's disease

Without special treatment, the patients will usually die after 7 to 10 years; in rare cases, after only 4 years; and in exceptional cases, after 20 years.

Prophylaxis and treatment of Alzheimer's disease

Attempts with vaccinations and immunosuppressive medicines:

Research is conducted for a vaccination with the target of stopping the disease. Unfortunately these efforts have so far not led to any results[143]. Research of a beta amyloid immunotherapy with the monoclonal antibody Bapineuzumab did not lead to any positive results either, and was discontinued. Further research with the monoclonal antibody 9D5 was successful in mice. It is targeted at the toxic protein pyroglutamate Abeta, which collects in the brains of mice in which Alzheimer's disease was artificially introduced. Results in humans are not yet established[144, 145].

The chemotherapeutic Bexarotene was able to dissolve up to 75 % of the β-amyloid plaques in mice and reduce memory deficits of the animals[146, 147, 148]. However, these results could not be confirmed in subsequent examinations by other groups of researchers. Bexarotene is not approved for treatment of Alzheimer's disease.

Acetylcholinesterase inhibitors (galantamine, donepezil, rivastigmine, huperzine A) are medicines that inhibit the reduction of the neurotransmitter acetylcholine. Brain sections that are important for associative thinking work with acetylcholine. They activate the memory performance in the hippocampus. This explains why these medicines can activate the memory activity of the hippocampus[149]. These medicines are approved for treating mild to medium Alzheimer's dementia, although their effectiveness is disputed[150].

Non-steroidal antirheumatics (NSAR)
In retrospective studies, it was found that patients with rheumatism develop Alzheimer's dementia less often and at older ages[151]. This has led to the conclusion that this age difference is attributable to the rheumatism treatments (NSAR, non-steroidal antirheumatics) which the patients often follow for years[152, 153]. In some transgenic animal models, it could be shown that the administration of Ibuprofen slightly reduced the deposits of β-amyloid plaques[154, 155, 156]. There have been no randomised double-blind studies for humans that would confirm such an effect. Based on animal tests, it is suspected that very high dosages would be necessary, leading to massive side effects on long-term application.
Therefore prophylaxis or treatment of Alzheimer's disease with these medicines

is not recommended[157, 158]. Additionally, these medicines will promote cardiovascular problems if used in high dosages for long periods of time[159].
Nevertheless, there are currently several clinical studies on the application of Ibuprofen in Alzheimer's disease[160].

Diethylperazine and its derivatives
In animal tests, it was possible to slow down degeneration of the nervous system by activating transport systems by means of diethylperazine and related medicines. They are currently being tested in humans[161].

NMDA receptor antagonist
The messenger substance glutamate is the most important exciting neurotransmitter of the brain. It is involved in learning processes and memory functions. It is distributed in higher amounts in Alzheimer's dementia. The medicine Memantine is to normalise the glutamatergic signal propagation that is increased in Alzheimer's dementia. In clinical studies, a slight improvement of the mental disorder in Alzheimer patients with medium to severe symptoms could also be documented. This medicine is not approved for mild dementia, but only for moderately to severely affected patients[162].

Cannabis
A systematic overview paper from the Cochrane Collaboration, published in 2009, showed that cannabis does not positively affect Alzheimer's dementia at all. This was confirmed in 2016[163].

Insulin
Insulin applied as a nasal spray can slightly slow the progress of Alzheimer's disease. It is suspected that this is due to a direct effect via the olfactory cerebrum[164].

Ginkgo biloba
Ginkgo biloba as standardised extract EGb 761 at a dose of 240 mg/day is only approved for symptomatic treatment of Alzheimer's disease. Its effect was partially described as 'promising'[165]. Nevertheless, its effect is assessed, with various interpretations[166].

Vitamin E
Vitamin E at high doses can slow the onset of requiring nursing[167].
The medicine Memantine disappointed in the same randomised study. The Alzheimer's Disease Cooperative Study-Activities of daily living (ADCS-ADL-study) observed the daily practical skills. Administration of vitamin E was able to slightly delay the deterioration of such skills. Other studies on vitamin E at high doses led to highly contradictory results[168, 169, 170, 171]. Since the effect is very slight and there are indications that high vitamin E doses will increase the risk of death[172], this treatment is not recommended.

Green tea and black tea
Lab tests show that the antioxidant epigallocatechin gallate (EGCG) from green tea may inhibit the formation of amyloid plaques[173, 174]. Other lab experiments show that epigallocatechin gallate may also dissolve amyloid plaques[175, 176, 177].
In mice it was shown that the plaque burden on the cerebral cortex, the hippocampus and the entorhinal cortex (olfactory cerebrum) was reduced by 54 %, 43 % and 58 %, respectively, after treatment with highly dosed EGCG over a period of six months[178]. Another study is underway at the Charité Berlin[179]. Lab examinations were able to show that theaflavin shares of black tea also prevented the formation of plaques and were able to dissolve existing plaques[180].

Clinical studies with patients are still pending. The effect of these flavonoids with antioxidant effect indicate the great relevance of oxidative stress as a cause of amyloid formation in Alzheimer's disease and formation of α-synuclein in Parkinson's disease.

The officially recognised risk factors of Alzheimer's disease

They mostly correspond to those of other civilisation diseases, in particular cardiovascular diseases, arteriosclerosis, apoplexy and vascular dementia. They are still being weighted differently at the moment[181]. The effect of preventive medicines has not yet been proven clearly[182]. While there have been many observatory studies, there have not been enough controlled randomised studies. It has been documented, however, that hypertension undoubtedly creates a significant risk for developing Alzheimer's disease[183].

Order therapy for Alzheimer's disease

Pharmacologically therapeutic approaches are attempts to influence the inflammatory activity of the immune system in order to delay episodes of the disease, the progressive course and the final disaster of degeneration of the nerve axons. The treatment approach described in this book is very different, which is about tackling all the evident causes of this tragic disease, remedying them and supporting the regenerative forces. It is about the effect of a comprehensive causative treatment as described herein. Those who begin early may expect a significant delay, even a standstill in many cases, of the degenerative processes. In the early stage, mental abilities can often be regained when comprehensive treatment is performed consistently.

Dietary treatment of neurodegenerative diseases

Fresh, plant-based food (raw vegetarian food) is decisive for successful treatment because of the very order of its energy potential that can regenerate cells. The 'information' from sunlight that is absorbed through photosynthesis renews the LASER amplification in the genetic material, the DNA of the cells, so that its energy is and remains removed from the thermodynamic balance so that the second law of thermodynamics does not apply. The ordering, regenerating principle (Prigogine's coherence principle) prevails over Clausius' degenerating chaos principle.

A high proportion of fruit and vegetables in the diet is the most effective protection against degenerative conditions[301]. The recommendations of the German society for nutrition (deutsche Gesellschaft für Ernährung, DGE) have been adjusted as a result of this insight[184]. We refer here to Bircher-Benner manual no. 4: Manual of fresh juices, raw vegetables and fruit dishes.

The high content of pharmacologically active substances in raw food, the secondary plant substances (phytochemicals), and specifically those with antioxidative effects, are also very important. We have seen how much the oxidative stress from toxins, high-frequency radiation and an unhealthy lifestyle and nutrition contrary to the needs of our biological nature are the root cause of the harmful effects on the nerve cells (neurons) described above. The diet should have a very high antioxidative potential that is capable of capturing and neutralizing free radicals. Every vegetarian raw food dish has a high antioxidative potential if the plant from which it is derived is capable of performing photosynthesis. Plants with particularly strong antioxidative (and therefore regenerative) effects should be preferred. These are foods with a high content of flavonoids and carotenoids. Flavonoids are found in particular in the outer layers of fruits and vegetables. Therefore they are mostly lost when vegetables and fruits are peeled. The protective effect of the carotenoids (xanthines), however, is lost in cooking[302].

Carotenoids
These are the red and yellow pigments in fruits, roots, leaves and vegetables.
They fight cancer, modulate the immune system and achieve an antioxidative effect by neutralising free radicals. Free radicals are highly reactive disintegration products of the water or nitrogen-oxygen molecules that mutate healthy cells into cancer cells.

Oxygen-containing carotenoids are lutein, zeaxanthin and β-cryptoxanthin. They mostly occur in the yellow and red parts of plants and are relatively stable in heat, so that they remain effective when cooked. Lutein is particularly important for the retina in the eye, the cells of which are specialised nerve cells of the brain.

Oxygen-free carotenoids are lycopene, α-carotene and β-carotene. They occur mostly in the green parts of plants and are sensitive to heat. Therefore an essential part of the antioxidative effect of carotenoids that protects from cancer is lost when cooking green vegetables. Raw carrots and pumpkins are particularly rich in α-carotene. Apricots, green cabbage, spinach, pumpkins and carrots are particularly rich in β-carotene when not heated. Lycopene is found almost exclusively in tomatoes. Lutein and zeaxanthin, which are important for the retina, are found mainly in green cabbage and spinach, where cooking only destroys them very slightly. About 10 % of the carotenoids act as provitamin A, which is converted into the antioxidative active vitamin A.

Flavonoids
Flavonoids have an antioxidative effect. They are found in the outer layers of fruits and vegetables, but also in their leaves. Yellow flavonoids, as contained in yellow fruits and vegetables, have given these substances their name (flavus means 'yellow'). The flavonoid group of anthocyanin provides the red, yellow and violet colours, as in cherries, plums, berries, red cabbage and aubergines. The flavonoid quercetin is very common. Its glycoside (quercetin bound to sugar) is called rutin. Quercetin is common in yellow onions and (in descending order) green cabbage, green beans, apples, cherries and broccoli. Quercetin is metabolised by the intestinal flora. It destroys carcinogenic substances (carcinogens)[302].

Flavonoids are highly effective antioxidants. In addition, they are active against pathogens and cancer. Their ability to modulate the disturbed immune system concomitant with neurodegenerative diseases, as well as their anti-inflammatory effect in the cerebral immune system of the microglia, which maintains the destructive processes in the nervous system, are essential for preventing and healing such conditions. Flavonoids also regulate the permeability of the capillary blood vessels (vascular permeability)[301]. They supplement the effects of vitamin C.

Although flavonoids are not destroyed by cooking, they can be destroyed by storage. Stored winter apples contain 50 % of their flavonoids. In August, head lettuce and endives contain five times as many flavonoids as in April. Processed foods have about 50 % of the flavonoid content of freshly harvested fruits[186].

Polyphenols
These substances (phenols, phenolic acids, cumarins, flavonoids, isoflavonoids, lignans, lignins, etc.) are highly active antioxidants. They protect the outer layers of the plant, and thus its inner parts, against oxidation. Green cabbage, whole wheat grains, radishes and white cabbage are particularly rich in polyphenols, followed by green and other fruits, nuts and coffee beans. Carrots contain 85 % of their polyphenols in their skin, and wheat has the largest share in the bran. Wholemeal wheat contains 10 times more polyphenols than coarsely ground wheat flour. When stored, the polyphenols are gradually oxidised and lose their effect. If parts of a plant turn brown or black, the polyphenols are converted into toxic quinones by the enzyme phenoloxidase. Such parts are toxic and must not be eaten. The polyphenol ellagic acid induces (activates) detoxing enzymes in the intestinal mucosa (phase II enzymes) and thus reduces carcinogenic substances. Walnuts are particularly rich in ellagic acid, followed by fresh blackberries and raspberries, strawberries and pecan nuts. When cooking jam, three-quarters of the polyphenols in the berries are lost. Polyphenols are metabolised very quickly. Therefore fresh fruits, nuts and raw vegetables provide protection only if eaten several times a day, i.e. at each meal.

Protease inhibitors
These secondary plant substances split up proteins into amino acids. The protease inhibitors of the plants are chains of approx. 100 amino acids that are connected

by disulphide bridges (sulphur bridges). Protease inhibitors not only protect from cancer and diabetes, they also have an antioxidative and anti-inflammatory effect and thus counter degenerative processes. They are also very important for the prevention of and fight against neurodegenerative processes.

Protease inhibitors are contained in fresh soy beans, mung beans, garden peas, unroasted peanuts, potatoes, rice, corn, oats and wheat. They are shown to have an anti-carcinogenic effect in animal studies[187].

Terpenes
These are aromatics (smell and taste substances) of plants. The terpene limonene of lemons increases the activity of detoxification enzymes in the small intestine and the liver, including glutathione-S-transferase. Limonene and carvone from caraway are effective for combatting cancer[188] in animal experiments. Limonene, derived from the essential oil of lemons, is not toxic even at high doses. Therefore it is particularly suitable for fighting neurodegeneration and cancer.

Sulphides
The sulphur compounds of the sulphides are what give onion and garlic their typical smell. The volatile (pungent smelling) garlic oil consists of different allyl sulphides. The main effect of garlic is caused by allicin, its characteristic aromatic substance. Allicin has a strong protective effect against oxidation and against the effect of free radicals. This makes it particularly valuable for the prevention of and fight against neurodegenerative conditions.

Vitamins A, C, D, E, folic acid and *polyunsaturated vegetable oils.*
As we have seen, the blood levels of vitamins A, C, D and E are very important for the prevention and healing of neurodegenerative processes. Vegetarian fresh food is very rich in folic acid.

Vitamin B_{12} is highly relevant for the conversion of the precursors of folic acid into its active form. The vitamin B_{12} level must be closely monitored at regular intervals and restored to the upper standard limit, with sui-table preparations if necessary. Vitamins D and E are contained in cold-pressed vegetable oils such as sunflower oil, thistle oil, rapeseed oil, sesame oil, walnut oil, flaxseed oil, avocado, etc.

The polyunsaturated vegetable oils (PUFA) omega-3 and omega-6 act upon the immune system. Therefore it is very important to observe their ratios, since the ratio of omega-3 to omega-6 is often too low. Omega-6 vegetable oils have an antioxidative effect but stimulate inflammation processes, while omega-3 vegetable oils also have a strongly antioxidative effect but dampen the immune system. We have seen that excessive inflammatory processes in neurodegenerative diseases are very significant in relation to the degeneration of the nervous system. Therefore we recommend taking three tablespoons of flaxseed oil three times a day in any case. We have already explained why fish oils should no longer be used to supply omega-3 oils. Vitamin D is assimilated better when taken together with flaxseed oil.

A raw food vegetarian diet is very rich in vitamin C with its high bioavailability. The vitamin D level should be brought to the upper standard level through regular exposure to the sun (20 minutes per body side without sun blocker, but with the head covered, and not during the three hottest hours) and if necessary by taking suitable vitamin D preparations.

The intestinal flora and the enteral immune system

The effect of raw food for the restoration of the milieu in the gastrointestinal tract is very important. We have seen that the immune cells learn to acquire their immune competence, in the lymph cell nests of the intestinal mucosa (Payer's plaques) and to differentiate foreign, toxic, harmful substances and germs from the body's own useful and beneficial substances and germs; and that subsequently only approx. 10 % of them will migrate into the body as immunocompetent cells to assume their tasks there.

In all neurodegenerative diseases, but especially multiple sclerosis, autoimmune processes are closely involved in the destruction of the nervous system. Vegetarian food – especially when as fresh as possible – restores the milieu in the gastrointestinal tract in a relatively rapid and thorough manner. A vegetarian diet high in fresh raw food slowly replaces with aerobic, healthy intestinal bacteria the germs growing anaerobically that produce putrefaction toxins and that have developed in an environment of high-protein nutrition. The miscolonisation reduces and disappears entirely within a few months. Now immunocompetent lymph cells are developed again. This reliably reduces the autoimmune processes and finally brings them to complete halt, so that the inflammatory processes in the nervous system subside. Refer to the Bircher-Benner manual no. 14 for patients with gastrointestinal conditions.

Lab control recommendations for the attending physician during the diet

Before beginning the diet: complete blood count, ESR, CRP, homocysteine, Na, K, selenium, zinc, serum-albumin, GOT, GPT, pancreas amylase, LDH, vitamins A, D and B_{12}, TSH. We recommend regularly monitoring the levels of vitamins B_{12} and D and consistently replacing them to the upper standard level during the treatment.

Table on the effects of foods on neurodegenerative diseases

	Antioxidative and antidegenerative effect	Inhibition of inflammation	Immunomodulation
apple	+++[u]	++[u]	+++[u]
apricot	+++	+++	++r+
aubergine	+++	+++	+++
avocado	+++		+++
beetroot	+++	+++	+++
berry	+++	+++	+++
blueberry	+++	+++	++++*
bran	+++		
cabbage	++++	+++	+++
carrot	+++++	++[u]	+++++[u, raw]
celery/celeriac	+++		+++
chickpea			
citrus fruit	+++		+++
coconut	++++	+++	+++
corn	+		
cress	+++		
cucumber	+++	+++	+++
fennel	+++	+++	+++
flaxseed oil, flaxseed[raw]	+++++++[lip]	+++++[lip]	+++++[lip]
garlic	+++++[raw]	+++++[raw]	+++++[raw]
grape	+++	+++	+++
grapefruit	+++	+++	+++
horseradish[raw]	+++	+++	+++
kiwi	+++	+++	+++
leafy salad	+++		+++
leek	+++		
lettuce	+++	+++	+++
lychee	+++	+++	+++
mango	+++	+++	
melon	+++	+++	+++
nut	+++		++++
onion	+++[raw]	++++[raw]	++++[raw]
papaya	+++	+++	+++
passion fruit	+++	+++	+++
pear	+++	++[u]	+++[u]
pepper	+++	+++	+++

	Antioxidative and antidegenerative effect	Inhibition of inflammation	Immunomodulation
plant oil, poly-unsaturated (PUFA)	+++++	+++++[lip]	+++++[lip]
pomegranate	+++	+++	+++
potato	+++	++[raw, m]	+++
pulse	+++		++++
pumpkin	+++		
radish types	++++		+++
soy	++[raw]		++++[raw]
spinach	+++[raw]		+++
stone fruit	++++	+++	+++
tomato	+++[raw]	++[raw]	+++[raw]
wholegrain cereal	+++		++[raw]

u: The polyphenols are in the skins of fruit and vegetables, which therefore should not be peeled. Approx. 50 % of the benefits are lost when fruit and vegetables are stored.

lip: Oils with polyunsaturated fatty acids (PUFA) e. g. flaxseed, sunflower, sesame, nut, sunflower, rapeseed, grapeseed, etc., must never be heated. Flaxseed oil must be stored in a cool, dark place. Olive oil contains mostly monounsaturated fatty acids and therefore may be heated to 170°C. Flaxseed oil moderates the immune system and therefore counters inflammation. A 1:1 ratio of omega-6 oil to omega-3 oil is the target for dietary treatment of neurodegenerative diseases.

Table on the general effect of raw food therapy

This table shows general indications and effects that can be considered in treatment:

Preparation	Treatment	Effect	Duration	Quantity
Juice: fruit, raw vegetables, plant milk (almond soy, sesame), certified raw milk, if prescribed: additions of wholegrain cereal or flaxseed gruel (always ⅓ of the juice) or cream and a touch of lemon juice	general metabolism overload (fasting indication), obesity, heart and circulatory failure, gastrointestinal inflammation, kidney and liver inflammations, acute flu (fever)	detoxifying, relieving, dehydrating (relieves heart and circulation), seals vessels, reduces inflammation, deacidifying, promotes nutritional economy, restores the intestinal milieu, reduces weight	1–28 days depending on medical prescription for longer fasting treatments: 1–3 days	600–800 g fresh juices (3–4 glasses) 450–500 g plant milk or herbal tea, 200–400 calories

Preparation	Treatment	Effect	Duration	Quantity
Pureed (slightly greater quantity, oil added): fruit and vegetables mixed in the blender (vegetables with sauce, see recipes), plant milk (almond, soy, sesame), certified raw milk, sour milk, butter milk, whey, yoghurt	inflammations in the digestive system, convalescence	same as under 'juice', plus cellulose content (stimulation of the peristaltic), addition of oil	3–14 days depending on medical prescription	approx. 1200 calories (see daily menu)
Finely chopped: fruit and vegetables, finely cut, chopped (for sauces, see the recipe section) walnuts, almonds, hazelnuts finely ground; addition: plant or certified raw milk, buttermilk, sour milk, whey, yoghurt wholemeal grain: finely chopped or sprouted	as under 'pureed' further convalescence	as under 'pureed': fermentative peristaltic effect by cellulose in coarser form, more volume, higher saturation form, stimulation of the intestine	3–21 days depending on medical prescription	800–1200 calories see daily menu
Normal raw vegetables: fruit and vegetables whole or chopped (Bircher muesli) normally prepared (see recipe section) walnuts, almonds, hazelnuts, pine nuts (whole). Wholegrain: chopped, coarsely ground or in flakes. Certified raw milk raw, buttermilk and sour milk, whey, yoghurt	general realignment of the metabolic reaction obstipation eczema and any allergic diseases, migraine acne, furunculosis, chron. infection and susceptibility to infection, arteriosclerosis, hypertension, preparation and aftertreatment of surgery, rheumatism	can be applied for week and months, forces increased chewing as a coarser form and stimulates the saliva glands, mechanical cleaning of the teeth	on average 1–6 weeks or 1–3 days per week alternating with juice fasting, raw food with additions (see p. 76)	1200–1700 calories see daily menu

Practical application of the raw food therapy

When there is no question of kidney failure, it is usually best to begin the diet with the first diet level (the fresh juice and plant milk diet), since this will convert the metabolism and intestinal milieu the fastest. The patient will not feel hungry. See Bircher-Benner manual no. 4 on fresh juices, raw vegetables and fruit dishes, which should be read before starting the diet. After a patient-specific duration, it can be replaced by the second diet level (the vegan raw food diet). After the disease has developed, this diet form is the most effective. It can and should be continued for many weeks. Later the third diet level can be used, e.g. on weekends, with one-third hot meals. A cyclical approach has also proven to be valuable, e.g. using level I on Monday, level II during the week and level III on the weekends. The following menus and recipe suggestions have proven their worth for decades and have been designed in accordance with this procedure.

Menus

Menus for various raw food regimes

Fresh juice fasting (bed/juice day)
Morning and evening: 200 g fruit juice
Lunch: 200 g fruit juice or 200 g vegetable juice (tomato or carrot juice, or a mix of tomato, carrot and spinach juice)
Depending on the season:
orange and tangerine juice
grapefruit juice
berry juices
grape juice
plum juice
peach juice
apricot juice
Japanese persimmon (kaki) juice
apple and pear juice (fresh)

These juices can also be combined (e.g. berry with peach or apricot juice, apricot with orange juice, apple with pear juice).

Depending on doctor's orders, fresh juice fasting may be undertaken for one or several days – even two, three or (rarely) four weeks. Medical supervision during fasting and subsequent recuperation is important (see table on page 70, 71). If only mild effects of fasting are desired – in the sense of general detoxification, dehydration and rejuvenation – a strict fruit juice day can be used once a week within the raw food treatment or regular diet where complete rest (preferably bed rest) is possible. If you do not rest during the first one or two fasting days, the full effect will be impaired by fatigue and hunger, and there will not be proper relaxation and urine flow. Do not be deterred by reactions such as headache, nausea, pain in the limbs, and weakness (especially in the afternoon). These show that the body is doing its detoxification work during juice fasting, so that such days have meaning and purpose. Be sure to report your observations to your doctor.

2. Juice only day
High quality, relatively nutritious food is administered. This regime can be maintained for one week or longer with the addition of cereal gruels, and can be prolonged for several weeks with the avoidance of strong physical and mental stress. Juice only periods are suitable to start readjustment treatment, for dewatering and weight loss treatments or, if the organism is very low in respect of vital substance (e.g. in the case of chronic digestive diseases if a traditional bland raw food free diet has been administered). In such cases, fruit juice should initially be taken with $1/3$ flaxseed, barley or rice gruel. For dehydration treatments, urine and weight must be measured at regular intervals. If necessary, diuretic tea (solidago, rosehip) should be drunk.

Morning: 200 g fruit juice
150 g almond milk or yoghurt
1 cup of rosehip tea
Lunch: 200 g fruit juice
150 g almond milk or yoghurt
150 g vegetable juice

Evening: same as morning.

3. Fruit fasting days
Fruit fasting may replace juice fasting in bed (the strict form of the fruit juice fasting day), e.g. when metabolism change and stimulation of the intestine with cellulose content is the principal aim, rather than protection through free cellulose. Since this diet produces a strong feeling of satiation, fruit fasting can be performed even on days without complete rest, and for extended periods of time. However, the effect of juice fasting is more intense. Fruit fasting is indicated for persons with heart disease, chronic liver weakness, or lazy bowels. Other indications are an apple day for acute diarrhea and a strawberry day for celiac disease and abdominal congestion. Duration 1–5 days (longer if prescribed by the doctor).

Daily menu: 3 times 200–250 g (up to 300 g) washed, fresh, completely ripe, unsweetened fruit, e.g. berries, citrus fruit (oranges, grapefruit, tangerines), grapes, figs, melons, Japanese persimmons (kaki).

Special fruit fasting forms
Apple day: 5–6 times 1 large apple finely grated for acute gastrointestinal catarrh with diarrhoea.

Strawberry day: 3–4 times 200–250 g very ripe strawberries, unsweetened, for celiac disease (special form of chronic diarrhoea) and vitamin C deficit.

Blueberry day: 3 times 200–250 g blueberries for slight intestinal infection. Slightly constipating.

Blackberry day: 3 times 200–250 g completely ripe blackberries. Particularly rich in natural sugar and vitamin C. Nutritious and easy to digest.

Currant day: 3 times 200–250 g ($2/3$ red and yellow, $1/3$ black). For patients with liver problems particularly refreshing and thirst-relieving. Rich in vitamin C.

Japanese persimmon (kaki) day: 2 small (or 1 large) Japanese persimmon fruits, 4 times a day. Very nutritious and rich in vitamins C and B.

Grape day (traditional grape treatment): 750–1000 g sun-ripened grapes, if possible untreated, distributed over 4–5 meals per day. Wash thoroughly and remove any treatment residue (briefly wash in hot water). Eat whole fruit. Low in vitamins but particularly nutritious because of its high fruit sugar content. Liver protection. Stimulates intestine with seeds. Duration: 1–2 weeks, longer if prescribed by doctor (up to 6 weeks).

Fig day: 3 times 200 g fresh figs. Stimulates the intestine. Nutritious. No more than 1 day.

4. Raw vegetable menus
Below are seven examples of raw vegetable combinations for lunch for each season. (Special value is placed on the harmonious distribution of bulb, root and leaf raw vegetables, but always use them fresh and very ripe.) For a full daily menu, see page 74.

a) Spring:
1st day: fruits – nuts (also dried fruit) – radishes – fennel – head lettuce
2nd day: fruits – nuts – celery root/celeriac – tomatoes – cress
3rd day: fruits – nuts – carrots – chicory/endive – head lettuce
4th day: fruits – nuts – radish – lettuce – cress

5th day: fruits – nuts – beetroot – dandelion – head lettuce
6th day: fruits – nuts – cauliflower – spinach – cress
7th day: fruits – nuts – kohlrabi – tomatoes – head lettuce

b) *Summer:*
1st day: fruits – nuts – radish – tomatoes – head lettuce
2nd day: fruits – nuts – carrots – courgettes – head lettuce
3rd day: fruits – nuts – cauliflower – radishes – head lettuce
4th day: fruits – nuts – kohlrabi – cress – head lettuce
5th day: fruits – nuts – celery root/celeriac – lettuce – head lettuce
6th day: fruits – nuts – tomatoes stuffed with cauliflower – head lettuce
7th day: fruits – nuts – small carrots – cucumbers – head lettuce

c) *Autumn:*
1st day: fruits – nuts – celery root/celeriac – tomatoes – endives/chicory
2nd day: fruits – nuts – beetroot – sweet peppers – head lettuce
3rd day: fruits – nuts – black salsify – spinach – head lettuce
4th day: fruits – nuts – cauliflower – lamb's lettuce – endives/chicory
5th day: fruits – nuts – small carrots – courgettes – cress
6th day: fruits – nuts – radish – tomatoes – head lettuce
7th day: fruits – nuts – celery root/celeriac – cucumbers – head lettuce

d) *Winter:*
1st day: fruits – nuts – black salsify – red cabbage – endives/chicory
2nd day: fruits – nuts – celery root/celeriac – radicchio – head lettuce
3rd day: fruits – nuts – carrots – sweet pepper – head lettuce
4th day: fruits – nuts – beetroot – sauerkraut – endives/chicory

5th day: fruits – nuts – cauliflower – spinach – lamb's lettuce
6th day: fruits – nuts – tomatoes – chicory/endive – head lettuce
7th day: fruits – nuts – celery root/celeriac – Savoy cabbage – chicory/endive

Daily Menu

Breakfast

Bircher muesli	120–200 g
ground almonds or hazelnuts	20–30 g
fruits	100–200 g
optional rosehip tea	1 cup

If a mushy or liquid consistency is desired: Bircher muesli with finely ground or mixed fruits (with crème, optional, 100–200 g), almond milk (20–30 g almond puree), 150 g fruit juice and 1 cup of rosehip tea.
The quantities need only be approximate to those indicated. What is important is the natural feeling that must not be impaired by stimulants or habits. Only where very little nutrition is desired should hunger be reduced by long chewing and salivation and by a slower intake of food.

Lunch

fruits or chilled fruit soup	150–250 g
green lettuce	50–100 g
raw vegetable plate	approx. 100–150 g
nuts of all kinds	approx. 20 g
1 glass of unfermented apple or grape juice (optional)	200 g

or

fruit juice	approx. 100–200 g
green lettuce, finely chopped	approx. 50 g
raw vegetables blended or mashed (cucumbers, tomatoes)	100 g
vegetable juice (spinach, carrots, etc.) with a touch of cream and lemon juice	100 g

almond milk or sesame milk approx. 200 g
apple or grape juice (optional)   200 g

Dinner
Bircher muesli   150–200 g
nuts   20–30 g
fruits   100–200 g
optional rosehip tea   1 cup

or
Bircher muesli   150–200 g
almond milk   approx. 200 g
fruit juice   approx. 200 g
optional rosehip tea   1 cup

5. Temporary and regular food
When patients have not relapsed for at least one year, they can add one third cooked food to their raw food diet, starting out entirely vegan. After two years they may carefully and sparingly add dairy products and eggs. It is important that they use raw food phases in between at regular intervals.

In the chapter 'Recipes', foods that are not vegan are marked with a *.

Example for a temporary day
Morning and evening: Same as raw food day.

Lunch:
Fruits, nuts, raw vegetable plate, 2 dl vegetable bouillon,
2 baked potatoes (see recipe page 93)

Example for a normal diet day
Breakfast:
Bircher muesli with ground nuts,
2 slices of wholemeal bread or crispbread,
approx. 15 g butter (optional)
fruits
herbal tea, or milk or yoghurt

Lunch:
fruits
raw vegetables: cauliflower, spinach, head lettuce
potato soup
steamed tomato, vegetables
wholegrain rice with fresh butter only, no cheese, lightly salted

Dinner:
Same as breakfast, optional rosehip jam or honey as bread spread.

The Recipes

Recipes marked * are not vegan. They must only be used in the menu plan after two years without a relapse. Individual non-vegan ingredients that can be left out or replaced are also marked with an *.

Juices

Juices are from raw fruits and vegetables in a mechanically refined form, used as additional special enrichment, when coarse food (cellulose) is not permitted. Whole raw vegetables are always higher in their nutritional quality and cannot be permanently replaced by juice.

For the preparation of juices, raw vegetables must be cleaned thoroughly, pressed with a hand press or an electric centrifugal juicer, and served immediately. Letting them stand reduces their value.

If a small hand press is used, fruits and vegetables must be chopped. Grate apples, pears and all bulbous vegetables finely; chop leafy vegetables and herbs finely.
High quality grape, fruit and vegetable juices are available at health food stores.

Fruit juices
Unmixed fruit juices (without any additives): Orange, tangerine, grapefruit, apple, pear, grape, strawberry, blueberry, currant, cassis, raspberry, peach, apricot, plum, mango, Japanese persimmon (kaki), kiwi.

Mixed fruit juices: For example orange, tangerine, grapefruit, Japanese persimmon (kaki) or berry juice with apple juice or berry juice with peach, apricot or plum juice or whipped bananas with orange, berry, peach, mango or apricot juice. Additions to taste or as needed: lemon juice, honey, maple syrup, fruit concentrate, cream, yoghurt, almond milk (only to be used if patient also suffers from stomach complaints), flaxseed, rice or barley gruel.

Vegetable juices
When fresh they have a high mineral and vitamin content. Each juice has its own special value.

Unmixed vegetable juices: tomato, carrot, beetroot, radish, cabbage, celery root/celeriac, potatoes, all leaf, bulbous and root vegetables; stinging nettle, sorrel and dandelion juice for springtime blood-cleansing treatment.

Mixed vegetable juices: carrot, tomato, and spinach in equal proportions (very good flavour), tomato and carrot, tomato and spinach.
Other mixes (and cocktails) can be combined according to taste.
For variety, add sorrel, stinging nettle, chives, parsley, onions, tender celery leaves or roots, and other herbs.
Additions per glass (1 $^{1}/_{2}$ – 2 dl): a touch of lemon juice, fruit concentrate (optional, small quantity). Flaxseed (optional), rice or barley gruel. Other leafy vegetables or lettuces may also be used, such as white cabbage, cabbage, head lettuce, endives/chicory, lamb's lettuce, lettuce, dandelion.

Potato juice
Prepare scrubbed, peeled (optional) potatoes (do not use potatoes that are unripe, green or sprouted) as for carrot juice. Not very agreeable and only to be used on doctor's orders.

Gruel to accompany juices
The gruel is added to raw juices; in a proportion of 1/3 it neutralises the sharpness of the fruit or vegetable flavour. Only to be used if the patient also suffers from stomach complaints. The daily ration can be prepared once a day and kept in a Thermos flask.

Rice or barley gruel: Stir 1 heaped teaspoon of rice or barley wholemeal flour with 2 dl cold water and boil for 5 minutes, stirring constantly. Let cool.

Flax seed gruel: Rinse 1 tablespoon flaxseeds, boil in 2 dl water for 10 minutes, strain and let cool.

Bircher muesli

All recipes are for 1 person.

Apple muesli
In our long experience, the original apple muesli as invented by Dr Bircher and used successfully thousands of times with his patients has remained the best food for the regime.

Sweet-tart juicy apples with white flesh are best for muesli (e.g. Klar, Gravenstein, Sauergrauech, Menznauer Jäger, Jonathan, Ontario, Rubinette, Glockenäpfel, Braeburn, Topas, Champagner-Reinetten, Cox's Orange).

The flavour of drier apple types with a blander taste can be enriched with a pinch of the freshly grated peel of untreated oranges or lemons, or with orange juice, a little rosehip paste or freshly grated ginger.

Apple muesli with yoghurt, sour milk or buttermilk*
1 tbs oat flakes
3 tbs water
1 tbs lemon juice
2 tbs Bifidus yoghurt,
Bifidus sour milk or buttermilk
1 tsp honey
200 g apples
1 tbs hazelnuts or almonds, ground

Soak the oat flakes for 12 hours (overnight if for breakfast). Mix the oat flakes, yoghurt (or sour milk) and honey until smooth. Remove stems and calyxes from the washed apples and, using the Bircher grater, grate the apples into the sauce. Stir several times to keep the muesli attractively white. Spread the nuts on it and serve at once. Eat immediately.

Other versions: Replace oat flakes with wheat, rice, barley, rye, semolina, buckwheat or soy flakes, optionally mixed with yeast flakes (enriching the muesli with vitamin B).

Different version: Mix 1 teaspoon soaked oat flakes with 1 teaspoon cereal grains (soak in water for 24 hrs., then put through a sieve and rinse with cold water). Whole, chopped or mixed.

Apple muesli with almond or sesame puree (vegan) (basic recipe)
1 tbs oat flakes
3 tbs water
1/2 tbs lemon juice
1 tbs almond or scsame puree
1 tbs honey
3 tbs water
200 g apples
1 tbs hazelnuts or almonds, ground

Soak oat flakes for 12 hours. Stir in lemon juice, puree, honey and water with a whisk to produce a creamy consistency, add the oat flakes and apples (prepared like basic recipe). Spread the nuts on top and serve at once.

Apple muesli with cream*
(Specially enriched recipe designed for weight gain. For diabetics, no honey or oat flakes. For diabetics with a low-fat diet, with unsugared condensed milk.)
1 tbs (8 g) fine oat flakes
3 tbs water
½ tbs lemon juice
3–4 tbs cream
1 tbs honey
200 g apples
1 tbs hazelnuts or almonds, ground

Prepared as for basic recipe.

Muesli with berries and stone fruit
Rich in vitamin C.
Prepare an almond puree, sesame puree or yoghurt dressing.
Add 150–200 g strawberries or raspberries, blueberries, currants or blackberries, and mash slightly with a fork.
Or
150–200 g plums, peaches or apricots, pitted and passed through the chopper or cut finely with a knife.

Bircher muesli with various fruits
The following combinations are very tasty:

strawberries and raspberries
strawberries, raspberries and currants
strawberries and apples
blackberries and apples
apples with finely cut orange and tangerine segments
apples and bananas
apples and peaches
sauce: almond or sesame puree sauce, or yoghurt dressing
Use only fresh fruits, never use canned fruits (fruit salad, etc.).

Muesli with dried fruits
If you have no fresh fruits at hand, you can also make the muesli with dried fruits (apples, apricots, plums, pears). One hundred grammes of dried fruits are washed, soaked in cold water for 12 hours and passed through the chopper. Mix with almond or sesame puree sauce or yoghurt dressing. For dried fruits, always look for good quality without preservatives or bleach; otherwise, gastrointestinal problems may occur.

Muesli with condensed milk*
If you do not have almond or sesame puree or fresh yoghurt at hand, you can make the muesli with condensed milk according to the original recipe. Disadvantage: Condensed milk often contains sugar.

Fruit and fresh grain dishes

Fresh grain cereal mash with banana
2 tbs cereal meal
½ banana
1 tsp honey
lemon as desired

Soak chopped cereal for 12 hours, then mix. Crush the banana with a fork and add it. Flavour with honey and lemon juice. Serve at once.

Fresh whole grain with berries
1 level tbs freshly ground wholemeal grains (wheat, rye, oats)
1 tbs water
1 tbs honey
lemon juice as desired
100 g berries (any kind)

Soak wholemeal grains for approx. 6 hours. Crush berries with a wooden spoon or mix with honey and lemon juice and mix into the grains.

Fresh whole grain with orange juice

1 level tbs freshly ground wholemeal grains (wheat, rye, oats)
1 tbs water
1 tbs honey
1 dl orange juice
1 tbs ground nuts

Soak wholemeal grains for approx. 6 hours. Mix in honey, orange juice and nuts.
The fresh, unblended whole grain can also be soaked and mixed in.

Sprouted cereal grains

These are very high in the vitamin E and B group, and generally have a strengthening effect.
1st day, evening: Wash the grains in a colander under running water and place them in a bowl. Cover with water and keep at room temperature, close to the oven.
2nd day, morning: Rinse the grains and spread to dry on a flat plate. Keep at room temperature, close to the oven.
Evening: put the grains back in the bowl and cover with water. Keep at room temperature, close to the oven.
3rd day, morning: Rinse the grains and spread to dry on the plate.
Evening: put the grains back in the bowl and cover with water. Keep at room temperature, close to the oven.
On the 4th day, the grains should have developed sprouts 1–2 cm long and are ready to eat.

The preparation of sprouted cereal grains is easier to accomplish in the practical sprouting devices that are available in various sizes.
Sprouted cereal grains are suitable to prepare muesli but also as an addition to salads or raw vegetables.

Chilled soups

Chilled soup

1 tbs honey
1 tsp agar-agar powder
1–1.5 dl water
2 peaches
or berries
or stone fruit
or pomes

Cook honey with agar-agar until the powder has completely dissolved. Cut the peaches finely and pour lemon juice over them to keep them from turning brown. Leave the berries whole, chop stone fruit or pomes.
Pour the sauce over the fresh fruit and allow it to cool.

Milk types

Almond milk

This food provides vegetable protein and oil and is rich in valuable unsaturated plant oils.
Stimulates mucous production and is soothing.

1 tbs almond puree
1 $\frac{1}{2}$ tsp honey
1 $\frac{1}{2}$ dl water and
and $\frac{1}{2}$ dl fruit juice (thickens slightly)

Whisk almond puree and honey and add the water drop by drop. Add the fruit juice last.

Almond milk of fresh almonds

Very easy to digest.

1 $\frac{1}{2}$ tbs almonds, peeled (no bitter almonds)
1 tsp honey
1 $\frac{1}{2}$ dl water

Mix almonds, honey and water in the mixer. Strain if necessary.

Pine nut milk
Very rich in easily digestible vegetable oils and protein that protects the metabolism.

1 1/2 tbs pine nuts, washed
1 tsp honey
1 1/2 dl water

Prepare as for almond milk.

Sesame milk
Rich in high-quality fatty acids.

2 dl water (cold or warm)
1 level tbs sesame puree
1 tsp lemon juice
1 tsp honey

Whisk almond puree and honey and add the water drop by drop. Add the lemon juice last.

Sesame cream
Like sesame milk, but with less water added. Replaces cream in cooked dishes and desserts.

Sesame frappé (milkshake)
Like sesame milk or sesame cream, with addition of fruit juice, apple juice, fruit concentrates.

Soy milk
1 cup soy beans
7 cups water
1 tbs fruit sugar
water

Wash and dry soy beans and grind them in an almond mill. Soak for 2 hours then boil for 20 minutes in the water used for soaking, stirring constantly. Strain. Add water until the viscosity of cow's milk is reached. Add fructose and let cool. Soy milk is sold in tetra packs in health food stores.

Raw vegetables and salads

There are three conditions to be respected when preparing raw vegetables and salads:

1. Freshness and quality
For any other diet and for full everyday nutrition, use only sunripened, organically grown vegetables and salads. They are not only ideal for health, but also taste best. Today the offer from businesses run in accordance with organic guidelines is very extensive, and organically grown vegetables are available in many supermarkets. Vegetables and salads from your own garden are, of course, ideal. Herbs and tomatoes can be grown even on a balcony. Choose young, tender leafy lettuces and root vegetables, unblanched, and remove any wilted leaves or rotting stalks. For a healing regime it is important to use only entirely fresh plants of the best quality. Prepare raw vegetables just before mealtime then mix them immediately with the dressing. Unless ingested immediately, chopped vegetables and salads rapidly lose their vitamin content.

2. Cleanliness
Vegetables grown organically without the use of artificial fertilizers contain no worm eggs. Nevertheless, all fresh plants must be cleaned thoroughly and carefully. Observe that water soluble substances such as Vitamin C, vitamins of the B group and minerals are leached out in water.

3. Harmonious composition
Every salad dish should contain all three types of vegetables: root, fruit and leaf. Green leafy lettuce in particular is always part of a healing regime. In the dressings, variety is desirable for the different ingredients of the raw food diet.
A beautifully assembled salad in pleasing colours is agreeable to the eye and the palate, and stimulates the appetite.
Small garnishes of herbs, radishes, young

carrots or olives make the raw vegetable dish even more colourful and festive. In everyday use the three kinds of vegetables per meal should not be exceeded. Too much variety may impair digestion.

Cleaning leafy vegetables
For head lettuce, endives/chicory, romaine lettuce, iceberg lettuce and similar green leaf lettuces, cabbage and red cabbage, etc. separate the leaves and clean them individually and carefully under running water. Rinse several times and dry thoroughly in a salad spinner.
Small-leaved salads such as lamb's lettuce and cut lettuce, spinach, dandelion, cress, rocket, radicchio and Brussel's sprouts should be rinsed repeatedly in small portions, and any hard stalks should be removed.
Halve chicory/endive and radicchio, remove outer leaves and rinse well.

Cleaning root vegetables
Celery root/celeriac, carrots, horseradish, radish, beetroot, kohlrabi, black salsify: clean with a brush under running water, peel and immediately grate or slice into the finished sauce. Mix well to preserve the vegetables' fresh colour.

Cleaning vegetable fruits
Wash tomatoes and cut them into wedges or slices. Peel cucumbers and cut them small or grate them. Organically grown young cucumbers do not need to be peeled.
Use only young, tender unpeeled courgettes for salads, wash them thoroughly, then slice or julienne them.
Green and yellow sweet peppers are milder than the red variety. Wash, halve, remove seeds and dice. Unfortunately, almost all non-organic sweet peppers now come from hydroponic production.
Separate cauliflower and broccoli into florets, and clean thoroughly under running water.

Wash stalk celery, peel when necessary, and cut away hard parts.
Halve leeks and fennel, prepare and wash under the spray tap.

Salad dressings

Use the various dressings as prescribed by a doctor.

Oil dressing (mild)
1 tbs oil (rapeseed, sunflower or olive oil from first cold pressing, thistle oil, walnut oil)
1 tsp lemon juice or organic fruit vinegar garlic, pressed
1 tsp fresh herbs (or 1 knife tip dried herbs)

Mix all the ingredients and whisk the dressing until creamy. The dressing also is even tastier with a splash of soy sauce or Kelpamare.
This classic salad dressing is suitable for all green salads (head lettuce, romaine lettuce, cress, etc.) and fruit salads (tomatoes, cucumbers etc.).

Quark dressing*
1 tbs lean quark
3 tbs butter milk
1/2 tsp fresh lemon juice
finely chopped herbs

Whisk all ingredients thoroughly.
This dressing goes particularly well with root vegetables (carrots, celery root/celeriac, radishes, etc.).

Yoghurt dressing*
For low fat diet.
2–3 tbs yoghurt
a few drops of lemon juice
onion, grated (optional)
a small amount of garlic, pressed (optional)
1 tsp fresh herbs (or 1 knife tip dried herbs)

Whisk all ingredients thoroughly.
A refreshing dressing with cress or spinach, with fruit salads (tomatoes, cucumbers) and with root vegetables (kohlrabi, horseradish, radishes).

Cream dressing*
2 tbs sour cream
1 tsp lean quark
1 tsp lemon juice
a small amount of pepper
1 tsp fresh herbs (or 1 knife tip dried herbs)

Whisk all ingredients thoroughly. This dressing goes well with almost all root and fruit salads. For a change, you may replace lemon juice with orange juice to give the raw food a new flavour. With celery root/celeriac, beetroot and chicory/endive salad, you may add a little freshly ground horseradish to this dressing for a very stimulating taste.

Almond puree or sesame puree dressing (mild)
1 tbs almond or sesame puree
3 tbs water
1 tsp lemon juice
a small amount of garlic, pressed (optional)
1 tsp fresh herbs (or 1 knife tip dried herbs)

Slowly stir sesame or almond puree with water until smooth, then add the other ingredients.
This tasty dressing is very suitable for root vegetables.

Classic mayonnaise recipe*
For 4 persons:
1 egg yolk
1 tbs lemon juice
2 dl oil
onion, herbs, a small amount of Kelpamare

Mix the egg yolk well with several drops of lemon juice. Add the oil drop by drop while whisking evenly. If the mayonnaise becomes too thick, dilute with lemon juice. Season to taste.

For 1 portion:
1 tbs mayonnaise
1 tsp lemon juice
1 tsp fresh herbs
(or 1 knife-tip of dried herbs)

Mix all ingredients well.

Mayonnaise with wholemeal soy flour instead of egg (mild)
For 6–8 portions.
2 tbs soy wholemeal flour
6 tbs water
2 dl oil

Mix soy wholemeal flour and water until smooth. Slowly add oil while constantly stirring with the whisk.
The mayonnaise can be kept in the refrigerator for a few days.

For 1 portion you need:
1 tbs mayonnaise
1 tsp lemon juice
a touch of mustard (optional)
1 tsp fresh herbs (or 1 knife tip dried herbs)

Mix all ingredients well.
Mayonnaise is a popular dressing for salads composed of field and root vegetables.

Raw vegetables, mixed
chicory/endive with diced tomato – oil dressing or mayonnaise
sweet pepper and fennel – oil dressing
fennel, chicory/endive, diced tomato – mayonnaise*
fennel and carrots – cream dressing or mayonnaise*
cauliflower and carrots – cream dressing or mayonnaise*
tomatoes and peppers – oil dressing

Tomatoes, raw, stuffed
with cucumbers – oil dressing
with celery root/celeriac – cream dressing*
with cauliflower – cream dressing*

Sauerkraut salad
Sauerkraut is a particularly wholesome raw vegetable, especially in winter. Sauerkraut is more easily digestible raw than cooked, and it has a gallbladder-purging and disinfecting effect. Use low salt organic sauerkraut if possible. An addition of finely-cut raw sauerkraut can considerably improve the taste and digestive qualities of steamed sauerkraut. For a salad, the sauerkraut is loosely separated and chopped, mixed with a few caraway seeds (or ground caraway), 3–4 chopped juniper berries, chopped onion, a julienned apple or a diced small fresh pineapple. Choose oil dressing as a dressing. This salad goes particularly well with corn salad and a raw root vegetable.

Mixed – pureed raw vegetables
If the doctor prescribes a 'pureed diet', certain raw vegetables may be mixed with the dressing in the blender. This is the transition from juice to normal raw vegetable food. The pureed vegetables must be eaten immediately after being spooned in and blended.

Examples:
1 tomato 70 g
1 handful head lettuce 30 g
1 small carrot 70 g
one knife tip marjoram
with oil dressing

1 tomato 70 g
1 handful head lettuce 20 g
1 small piece of celery root/celeriac 20 g
with oil dressing
(with lovage)

beetroot 30 g
zucchini 40 g
head lettuce 20 g
with cream dressing
(with dill)*

celery root/celeriac 40 g
carrots 40 g
spinach 20 g
almond puree dressing
(with rosemary)

Suggestions for dressings to go with the salads and raw vegetables

head lettuce	uncut	oil dressing	chives, onion
cut lettuce	uncut	oil dressing	chives, onion
chicory/endive	cut in strips of 1 cm	oil dressing	onion, parsley
lamb's lettuce	uncut	oil dressing	onion, parsley
cress	uncut	yoghurt dressing	chives
spinach	cut in strips of $1/2$ cm	yoghurt dressing	peppermint
cabbage lettuces: white cabbage, sauerkraut, Brussels sprouts, savoy cabbage	slice, cut into thin pieces	oil dressing or mayonnaise	lovage, savory, thyme, caraway
tomatoes	slice or dice	oil dressing or yoghurt dressing	basil, thyme, oregano
cucumbers	slice	oil dressing	dill

fennel	cut thin with knife	cream dressing or oil dressing	dill, chives, parsley
sweet pepper	cut into fine strips	oil dressing or mayonnaise	chives
radish	slice or grate	quark dressing	chives, parsley
radishes	slice or cut finely	yoghurt dressing	chives, parsley
stalk celery	cut finely	oil dressing or almond puree dressing	chives, thyme
courgettes	grate coarsely or slice	oil dressing or almond puree dressing	dill, borage, basil
carrots	grate finely	yoghurt or orange dressing	chives, lovage
celery root (celeriac)	grate finely	cream dressing	ginger
beetroot	grate finely	cream dressing	horseradish
cauliflower, broccoli	cut off florets, grate stems	garlic dressing	chives
endive/chicory	cut in strips of 1 cm	cream dressing	tarragon, parsley
Jerusalem artichoke	grate	mayonnaise	marjoram, thyme
kohlrabi	slice or grate	yoghurt dressing or cream dressing	thyme, lovage
red cabbage	slice or cut finely	almond puree dressing	grated apple, caraway, lovage

Chives, parsley and onions may be added in moderation to any raw vegetable, according to taste.

Cooked food

Such food is only used after the first healing phase, i.e. after the first two diet levels of raw food. Every meal must still begin with raw food. In particular in the summer months, when convenient, fresh juice and raw food days should also be used intermittently. The following cooked food should not make up more than one-third of the volume of the raw food eaten previously.

Recipes that contain animal protein and fat are marked with an asterisk (*). These may be used if one wants to prevent neurodegenerative diseases. However, someone who is suffering from a neurodegenerative disease should not use these recipes, since animal fats and proteins have to be avoided. Cream may be replaced by soy cream or a small amount of almond puree.

Garlic, a very important ingredient, is used mainly with raw food, since it loses much of its health-giving effect when heated, and the cooked recipes taste better with onions.

Every meal should begin with fruit and nuts. Breakfast and dinner should be small and as frugal as possible, as at the first and second raw food diet level.

One should drink only while eating the fruit, and repeatedly between the meals. Drinking with the fruit will send the fruit directly to the duodenum, which will promote digestion and development of the proper intestinal flora.

The recipes for cooked meals have been designed in accordance with the very valuable experience gained at the original Bircher-Benner medical centre. They appeal to the taste and are readily digestible. They correspond to a whole food diet as created by Dr. Maximilian Bircher-Benner, who also coined the term 'whole food'. The cooking times are indicated without the use of a pressure cooker or a steamer, and can be reduced to approx. one-third or one-fourth if such a device is used. This is highly recommended.

Recipes for cooked food

Soups
All recipes are for 1 person.

The following soup and vegetable recipes require a large amount of vegetable broth. In a small household, it is inconvenient to make fresh vegetable broth every day. Instead, you may use ordinary water and salt-free vegetable bouillon cubes or pastes.
In case of wheat allergy, the wholemeal flour in the recipes should be replaced by rice, millet or oat flour.

Vegetable broth
As the only exception, this recipe is for 4 persons.

1 tbs organic nut spread or olive oil
1 onion
2 carrots
1 small stalk of celery (150 g)
cabbage, Swiss chard leaves
1 leek stalk
3–4 l water
½ bay leaf
1 pinch rock salt
lovage, basil or
or other herbs, dried
or preferably fresh

Halve the onion, keeping the brown peel, and brown the cut area in the hot fat.

Chop the vegetables, add and cook for at least 15 minutes covered at low heat. Add water and cook for 2 hours at low heat. Season to taste.

Vegetable bouillon
3 dl vegetable broth
a pinch of rock salt (optional)
10 g nut spread or olive oil
parsley, chives, freshly chopped herbs

Prepare the vegetable broth according to the above recipe and add to nut spread, vegetable fat and herbs. Add more rock salt to taste.

Semolina dumplings*
10 g butter
1 ½ tbs fine semolina
½–1 egg
1 pinch rock salt
marjoram, nutmeg
6 dl vegetable broth

Cream the butter until foamy. Mix the semolina and egg thoroughly with the butter. Add salt and spices and let the mix stand for 30 minutes. Use a teaspoon to shape the dumplings. Place them in the boiling vegetable bouillon and steep for 15 to 20 minutes.

Rice soup, clear
½ tbs olive oil or organic nut spread
a small amount of chopped onion
1 small carrot
a small amount of celery root/celeriac and leek
1 tbs rice
1 pinch rock salt
6 dl vegetable broth
chives

Sauté onion with finely cut vegetables and rice. Add hot vegetable broth and cook for 15–20 minutes. Prepare with finely cut chives and vegetable fat.

Rice soup, thickened
1 tbs organic nut spread or olive oil
a small amount of celery root/celeriac
1 small carrot
a small amount of leek
1 tbs rice
½ tbs wholemeal flour
6 dl vegetable broth or water
lovage, parsley, basil, marjoram
a dash of soya sauce (optional)
½ tbs cream* or sesame cream (see recipe page 80)
chives

Sauté the chopped vegetables in the fat. Sprinkle with wholemeal flour, add the vegetable broth and cook for 30 minutes. Season with soy sauce and herbs. Place cream and finely cut chives in the soup bowl and serve the soup over them.

Oat cream soup
½ tbs organic nut spread or olive oil
2 tbs fine or coarse oat flakes
6 dl vegetable broth
a small amount of celery root/celeriac
½ tbs cream* or sesame cream (see recipe page 80)
optional: a small amount of miso, chives, nutmeg or caraway

Briefly sauté oat flakes with or without vegetable fat. Add vegetable broth and celery root/celeriac. Cook oat flakes for 10 minutes (coarse oats must cook for at least 20 minutes). Season to taste. Place cream or sesame cream and chives in the soup bowl and add the pureed soup.

Oat groat soup
½ tbs organic nut spread or olive oil
2 tbs oat groats
chopped onion
8 dl water or vegetable broth
a small amount of diced celery root/celeriac
1 pinch rock salt or a small amount of miso
chives, parsley, marjoram or borage

Sauté onion and groats with or without vegetable fat. Add vegetable broth and celery root/celeriac and cook for 45–60 minutes. Season to taste with a pinch of rock salt or miso. Place herbs in the soup bowl and add the soup.

Tomato soup
½ tbs organic nut spread or olive oil
a small amount of onion, celery root/celeriac and leek
1 small carrot
1 garlic clove
1 tomato
1 tbs soy wholemeal flour
6 dl vegetable broth
1 pinch rock salt
tomato puree (optional)
1 pinch fruit sugar
rosemary, oregano
5 g organic nut spread
½ tbs cream* or sesame cream (see recipe page 80)
chives

Sauté diced vegetables with or without vegetable fat, then add the tomato. Sprinkle with wholemeal flour and add vegetable broth. Cook for ½ hour then strain. Add spices and optional tomato puree. Place olive oil or nut spread and cream (optional) in the soup bowl, and add the finished soup. Sprinkle with finely cut chives. If desired, add 1 tablespoon rice to the soup or sprinkle with fat-free toasted bread cubes (croutons).

Summer tomato soup
4 ripe summer tomatoes
1 pinch fruit sugar
1 pinch rock salt
1 tbs cream* or sesame cream (see recipe page 80)

Dice the tomatoes, cook briefly, season and strain. Add the cream or sesame cream and serve the soup lukewarm or cold.

Vegetable soups carrots, spinach, broccoli, cauliflower)
½ tbs organic nut spread or olive oil
a small amount of chopped onion
1 ½ tbs wholemeal flour
1 pinch rock salt
6 dl vegetable broth
1 tbs cream* or sesame cream (see recipe page 80)
Vegetables: 1 diced carrot or 1 small cup of spinach pureed or finely chopped, broccoli or cauliflower finely chopped (cook some of the flowers separately and set them aside).

Sauté onion and carrots or broccoli with or without olive oil. Sprinkle with wholemeal flour and sauté them briefly. Pour in vegetable broth and cook for 20–40 minutes. For the spinach soup, add the spinach last and remove from heat. Pour the soup over the cream or sesame cream in the soup bowl. For the broccoli and cauliflower soup, add the flowers previously set aside.
Seasoning the vegetable soups: For carrot soup, use celery leaves or lovage, rosemary or marjoram, 1 teaspoon caraway. For spinach soup, use peppermint leaves, parsley, chives, one pinch of nutmeg. For broccoli or cauliflower soup, use a small amount of basil, parsley, chives, tarragon.

Chervil soup*
½ tbs organic nut spread or olive oil
a small amount of onion
1 medium-sized potato, chopped in cubes
½ tbs wholemeal flour
5 dl vegetable broth
1 pinch rock salt
1 tbs chervil, chopped
½ tbs cream* or sesame cream (see recipe page 80)

Sauté the onion slightly with or without vegetable fat. Add potato, sprinkle with wholemeal flour and add vegetable broth and a pinch of salt. Cook for ½ hour and strain. Put chervil and cream or sesame cream in the soup bowl and add the soup.

Potato soup
½ leek, cut into thin strips
½ carrot, sliced
½ tbs wholemeal flour
5 dl vegetable broth
1 medium-sized potato, diced
1 pinch stone salt or a small amount of miso
basil, marjoram
1 tbs cream* or sesame cream (see recipe page 80)

Sauté the leek and carrot in a little vegetable broth. Sprinkle with wholemeal flour and add the vegetable broth. Add potato and cook until soft. Season to taste. Place basil, marjoram and optional cream or sesame cream in the soup bowl and add the finished soup.

Minestrone
½ tbs organic nut spread or olive oil
2 tbs leek
a small amount of onion, finely chopped
a few celery leaves
½ plate mangold leaves
7 dl water or vegetable broth
1 tbs lovage or thyme
½ garlic clove, pressed
basil, parsley, chives
1 pinch rock salt
15 g pasta or rice
5 g nut spread or 1 tsp olive oil

Mince onion, leek, celery leaves and mangold leaves and sauté them slowly. Add vegetable broth, season and cook for 30 minutes. Add pasta or rice and cook another 15–20 minutes. To enhance flavour, add nut spread or olive oil.

Vegetables

Spinach, chopped

¼ l vegetable broth
200 g spinach (remove thick stems)
¼ garlic clove, pressed
1 pinch rock salt
peppermint leaves, sage
1 cup raw spinach
optional: fresh butter* or organic nut spread

Briefly cook spinach in the vegetable broth and drain, then cut, chop or blend. Return spinach to the pan and heat. Add garlic, salt and herbs. Chop or blend the raw spinach and add to the cooked spinach (with a little butter, olive oil or nut spread) before serving.

Spinach, whole leaves (and stems)

300 g spinach (remove thick stems, briefly boil the coarser winter spinach if required)
1 tbs pine nuts
1 tbs raisins (optional)
1 pinch rock salt
peppermint leaves, sage, parsley
optional: melted butter* or organic nut spread or olive oil

Sauté spinach uncovered over low heat with a little water. Add pine nuts, spices and optional raisins and briefly continue cooking. Add liquid butter, olive oil or nut spread to taste.

Lettuce

1 romaine lettuce
1 l water
a small amount of chopped onion
½ tbs organic nut spread or olive oil
1 dl vegetable broth
1 pinch rock salt
2 tbs cream* or sesame cream (see recipe page 80)

Halve the romaine lettuce, boil until softish then drain. Reassemble the lettuce and place in an oven-proof baking dish. Lightly sauté the onion with nut spread or olive oil and place it over the lettuce. Add vegetable broth and a pinch of rock salt and cook in the oven for 30–40 minutes. Add the cream or sesame cream 5 minutes before serving.

Sautéed chicory/endive

2 heads chicory/endive
½ tbs organic nut spread or olive oil
3 tbs vegetable broth
1 pinch sea salt
marjoram, thyme

Halve the chicory/endive and layer the leaves in the pan. Add heated nut spread or olive oil and vegetable broth to the chicory/endive, season and cook covered over low heat for 30 minutes. Spread melted nut spread or a little olive oil on the prepared vegetables.

Celery stalks

3–4 stalks celery
½ onion, chopped
a small amount of apple, finely chopped
1 dl vegetable broth
1 tsp almond puree
1 pinch rock salt or
a dash of soya sauce
celery greens

Cut the celery stalk into pieces 8 cm long and place in a pan. Briefly sauté the onion and apple without fat and spread over the celery. Add vegetable broth and almond puree and cook over low heat for ½ to ¾ hour. Season.

Baked fennel with cream cheese sauce*

1 large or 2 small fennel plants
1 pinch rock salt
pepper
several drops of lemon juice
1 cream cheese

Quarter the fennel and steam it until semi-soft. Pull apart the individual layers of the fennel bulb and place them in an oven-proof mould. Drizzle with lemon juice then add salt and pepper. Stir the cream cheese with 2 tablespoons of fennel stock and spread over the vegetables. Bake in hot oven.

Vegetable curry
1 tbs olive oil
1 spring onion
200 g vegetables (e.g. leeks, carrots, courgettes, asparagus)
½ tsp wholemeal flour
1 knife tip (to taste) curry powder
½ tsp vegetable broth
½ orange
1 tsp sultanas
1 pinch whole cane sugar
1 pinch rock salt, pepper

Cut the spring onion into fine rings and cook in slightly heated oil. Sprinkle on flour and curry powder and add the vegetable broth. Add the finely cut vegetables and cook covered for approx. 15 minutes. Set aside two or three wedges of the orange, squeeze the rest and place the sultanas in the juice. When the vegetables are soft, add the sultanas and orange juice, heat the mixture and season with sugar, salt and pepper. Serve and spread the orange wedges on top.

Cooked carrots
3–4 carrots
1 dl vegetable broth
1 tsp almond puree
1 pinch each fruit sugar and rock salt
marjoram, thyme, rosemary, parsley

Cut the carrots in strips or rounds and sauté in the vegetable broth for 30–45 minutes. Stir in the almond puree (optional). Season and sprinkle the chopped parsley.

Peas and carrots
½ tbs organic nut spread or olive oil
100 g fresh peas, shelled
1 dl vegetable broth
marjoram, thyme, lovage, parsley, chives
150 g sliced carrots, prepared according to the above recipe for cooked carrots

Briefly sauté peas in the nut spread or olive oil, add vegetable broth and cook until soft. Season. Mix carrots and peas or serve them alternately on the platter.

Cooked sugar peas (snow peas) (mange tout)
200 g snow peas
1 dl vegetable broth
1 pinch rock salt
1 pinch whole cane sugar
a small amount of parsley or lovage
organic nut spread or olive oil

Cook sugar peas and herbs covered in the vegetable broth for ½ to ¾ hour. Season and add olive oil or nut spread when serving.

Green beans with tomatoes
½ tbs organic nut spread or olive oil
½ onion
250 g beans
a small amount of garlic
savoury, parsley
1–2 tomatoes
1 pinch rock salt
caraway, marjoram, lovage

Sauté the chopped onions in organic nut spread or olive oil. Sauté the beans, finely diced tomatoes and herbs for approx. 1 hour. Add water if necessary. Season.

Steamed celery root/celeriac
½ tbs organic nut spread or olive oil
½ onion
½ celery root/celeriac
1 dl vegetable broth
1 pinch rock salt
a small amount of lemon juice, marjoram
1 tsp almond puree
very thin slices of apple, nuts

Sauté the chopped onions in organic nut spread or olive oil. Add the julienned celery root/celeriac and vegetable broth and cook until soft, $1/2$ to $3/4$ hour. Season. To refine, add almond puree and, if desired, apple slices. Sprinkle with chopped nuts.

Stewed tomatoes
4–5 tomatoes
$1/2$ tbs organic nut spread or olive oil
$1/2$ onion
fruit sugar
1 pinch rock salt
touch of garlic
rosemary, marjoram, basil
1 tbs maize flour (optional)
parsley or chives or dill

Slightly brown onion and fruit sugar in nut fat or olive oil in a frying pan. Douse the tomatoes with boiling water then peel them, cut them into pieces, add them to the onions and cook the mixture until slightly thickened. Add garlic and spices and finish cooking (add maize flour to thicken). Sprinkle chopped parsley or other herbs abundantly on the prepared tomatoes.

Baked tomatoes
2–3 tomatoes
1 pinch rock salt
10 g organic nut spread or olive oil
$1/4$ onion, chopped herbes de Provence (basil, rosemary, thyme, sage), parsley

Sauté the onion without fat. Put the halved tomatoes on a greased tray or ovenproof dish. Add dabs of nut spread or rub olive oil on each tomato half, and spread the sautéed onion and herbs on it. Cook briefly in the oven.

Some tomatoes may be minced or very finely chopped, blended with cream*, parboiled briefly and spread over the prepared tomato.

Tomatoes à la Provençale
2 tomatoes
1 pinch rock salt
1 tbs chopped parsley
1 tbs breadcrumbs

Halve tomatoes, sprinkle with rock salt, and place on a tray. Mix breadcrumbs and parsley and spread on the tomatoes with a spoon. Bake in the oven for 15 minutes.

Courgettes with tomatoes
$1/2$ tbs organic nut spread or olive oil
$1/2$ onion, chopped
300 g courgette
50 g tomato
1 pinch rock salt
garlic, rosemary, marjoram, thyme, basil, parsley, chives, dill
maize flour (optional)
1 tsp almond puree

Simmer onion in vegetable fat. Dice the courgettes; peel and dice the tomatoes. Add the vegetables to the onions and cook until soft. Season to taste. If there is too much liquid, add stirred maize flour and 1 teaspoon almond puree before serving.

Sweet peppers (green, yellow, red)
These are very suitable as an addition to other dishes.
150– 200 g sweet peppers
$1/2$ tbs organic nut spread or olive oil
$1/2$ onion, chopped
1 pinch rock salt
garlic, rosemary, marjoram, thyme, basil, parsley

Cut the sweet peppers in strips and sauté them in nut spread or olive oil with the onion, herbs and spices in a covered pan for at least $1/2$ hour.

Ratatouille
50 g sweet peppers
100 g courgette

50 g aubergine
1 tomato
½ onion, chopped
a small amount of garlic
1 tbs organic nut spread or olive oil
1 pinch rock salt
rosemary, marjoram, thyme, basil, parsley

Chop the sweet peppers, courgettes, aubergines and tomato (peeled). Sauté onion and garlic in nut spread or olive oil, add vegetables and cook covered for 1 hour. Season. If there is too much sauce, leave it to thicken while uncovered.

Aubergines
Wash the aubergines, peel (optional)
1 tbs organic nut spread or olive oil
400–500 g aubergines
a small amount of vegetable broth (optional)
rock salt
1–2 tomatoes

Steam the aubergines, cut into cubes, and sauté in nut spread or olive oil until soft. Salt as allowed. Garnish with a few tomato halves or with stewed tomatoes.

Artichokes
1 artichoke
¾ l water
1 tbs lemon juice
1 pinch rock salt

Cut off the stalks close to the artichokes themselves. Remove the bottommost hard leaves and remove the tips. Halve and cut out the heart; wash under running water and rub the cut surface with lemon juice. Bring water to the boil, add lemon juice and rock salt, and cook the artichoke until soft for approx. ¾ hour. Drain and serve the artichoke on a warm platter covered with a serviette.
Serve with vinaigrette (see recipe page 99).

Asparagus
¾ asparagus bunch
1 l water
1 pinch rock salt
a small amount of grated cheese*
nut spread or olive oil

Wash the asparagus and peel the stalks thoroughly. Green asparagus can be left almost whole. Cook the asparagus in boiling water for 20–30 minutes until soft (quicker with green asparagus), remove with a slotted skimming spoon and serve on a platter covered with a serviette. Sprinkle cheese* and pour liquid nut spread or olive oil over the dish.
As a variation, serve with vinaigrette sauce (see recipe page 99).

Cauliflower or broccoli
Only from organic production.
1 small cauliflower or broccoli (250 g)
1 tsp organic nut spread or olive oil
1 garlic clove
1 dl vegetable broth
1 pinch rock salt, pepper
pine nuts or almond slices

Cut off the leaves and stalk below the flower. Peel the stalk and cut into larger pieces; divide the flower into florets. Lightly brown the chopped garlic clove in nut spread or olive oil, add the cauliflower or broccoli and sauté briefly. Cover with vegetable broth and cook for approx. 5 minutes. Season with a pinch of salt and pepper. Briefly brown pine nuts or almond slices in a frying pan without fat and spread on the vegetables.

Cabbage or white cabbage, steamed
Do not eat cooked cabbage if you are suffering from flatulence. Cabbage does not cause flatulence when raw. All cabbages must be chewed well; raw cabbage juice is always permitted and does not cause flatulence.
½ tbs organic nut spread or olive oil
½ onion, chopped

250 g young cabbage
1 dl vegetable broth
nutmeg, caraway, 1 pinch rock salt
basil or lovage

Sauté onions in nut spread or olive oil. Cut cabbage in strips 2 cm wide, add to the onions and cook until the vegetables begin to soften. Add vegetable broth and cook over low heat for 30 minutes until soft. Season.
Green, mature cabbage must be blanched before cooking.

Red cabbage
Avoid if suffering from meteorism.
$1/2$ tbs organic nut spread or olive oil
250 g red cabbage
$1/2$ tbs lemon juice
$1/2$ apple
$1/2$ tbs rice
1 dl vegetable broth
$1/2$ dl grape juice or apple juice
1 apple
a small amount of butter*
1 pinch rock salt

Steam the finely grated red cabbage in vegetable fat. Add lemon juice, apple cut into fine slices and rice. Continue steaming. Add vegetable broth and grape juice or apple juice and steam until soft, covered over low heat for $1 - 1 1/2$ hours. Peel the second apple, cut into wedges. Add butter and braise the apple wedges on a tin baking sheet in the oven. Garnish the prepared red cabbage with the apple wedges.

Salads of cooked vegetables

Carrots, celery root/celeriac, beetroot, beans, cauliflower, broccoli, courgettes, mangold leaves and Swiss chard are particularly suitable for these salads.
The vegetables are cooked in vegetable broth or water until soft, drained and cut small (diced, sliced, florets, strips). Serve with salad dressing or with vinaigrette or mayonnaise. Enhance with onions and chopped herbs.

Potato salad
200 g potatoes
$1/2$ dl vegetable broth
1 tbs mayonnaise or
sesame mayonnaise (see recipe page 82)*
$1/2$ tbs chopped onions
borage, chives, parsley
lemon balm, marjoram, thyme, dill

Cook the potatoes until soft in the pressure cooker, peel while hot and slice. Pour the heated vegetable broth on them and let stand for a short time, then mix in the mayonnaise*. Season with onions and herbs. Mayonnaise can be replaced with oil, lemon juice and cream, well mixed and added to the potatoes.

Potato salad with cucumbers
1 large potato
$1/4$ cucumber
2 tsp yoghurt dressing (see recipe page 81)*
$1/2$ garlic clove
dill or borage, chives
parsley, onion

Prepare the potato as described above. Coarsely grate the peeled cucumber and add to the potato. Mix with yoghurt dressing and season with onions and herbs. Rub the salad bowl with the garlic clove before serving.

Salade niçoise*
1 boiled potato
1 small tomato
radishes
several cucumber slices
1 hardboiled egg*
1 tbs oil
$1/2$ tbs lemon juice
1 pinch rock salt
parsley, chives or dill

lemon balm, borage
a few leaves of head lettuce

Slice the potato, tomato, radish and egg and, together with the cucumber slices, top with a salad dressing of oil, lemon juice, rock salt and herbs. Just before serving, cut the leaves of head lettuce into broad strips and mix with the salad or prepare the salad on the head lettuce leaves.

Vegetable aspics
2 ½ dl vegetable broth
2 g agar-agar
a few drops of lemon juice
a pinch of rock salt
fresh slices of cucumber
cubes of tomato
broccoli flowers, cooked
peas, cooked
beans, cooked and finely chopped

Agar-agar is vegetable gelatine powder that is used for vegetable and fruit aspics, sauces and puddings, etc. instead of animal gelatine.
Add agar-agar powder to the lukewarm vegetable broth and heat slowly until the gelling agent is thoroughly dissolved. Season with lemon juice and a small amount of rock salt. Pour a little aspic into the rinsed moulds and let it harden. Garnish with vegetable slices, add more aspic, let it harden and repeat until the moulds are filled.
Turn over the cooled aspics and serve on a bed of salad leaves.

Potato dishes

Potatoes in their skins
3–4 small potatoes
water

Brush and wash potatoes. Fill pan with steamer insert or wire screen with water up to the insert, add potatoes, cover and cook for 30–40 minutes (8–10 minutes in the pressure cooker).

Baked potatoes (jacket potatoes)
3–4 small potatoes
1 tbs olive oil
butter*, nut spread or olive oil

Brush and wash the potatoes. Score the peel on the top 3–4 times, brush with oil and bake the potatoes on a greased sheet at medium heat for 30–40 minutes. Put a dab of butter* or nut spread on each of the cooked potatoes or brush with olive oil.

Caraway potatoes
2–3 medium-sized, longish narrow potatoes
1 tsp caraway
1 pinch rock salt
1 tbs olive oil

Wash and clean the potatoes and cut them in half crosswise. Mix caraway with rock salt and sprinkle on the cut side of the potatoes. Place the potatoes with the cut side down on a greased tray, brush with olive oil and bake at medium heat for ¾ hour.

Bouillon potatoes
250 g potatoes
1–2 dl vegetable broth
1 pinch rock salt
lovage, thyme
10 g butter*, organic nut spread or olive oil

Wash potatoes, peel, halve or cut into pieces and cook until soft in the vegetable broth with the salt and spices. Spread butter or nut spread on the prepared potatoes or brush with olive oil.

Potatoes with tomatoes
200 g potatoes
½ small onion
1 dl vegetable broth

1 small tomato
1 pinch rock salt
1 tbs cream* or sesame cream (see recipe page 80)
marjoram, rosemary or thyme

Briefly sauté the chopped onion and peeled, sliced potatoes without fat, then cook them in the vegetable broth until softish. Cut the peeled tomato into wedges, add and finish cooking. Season. Add the cream or sesame cream before serving.

Mashed potatoes
4 potatoes
water for steaming
dried tomatoes
butter* or organic nut spread or olive oil

Wash, peel, quarter and steam the potatoes until soft. Rice the potatoes onto a warm plate. Add liquid butter, nut spread or olive oil and garnish with minced dried tomatoes.

Roast potatoes
2 small potatoes
water for steaming
1 pinch rock salt
1 dl vegetable broth
1–2 tbs cream* or sesame cream (see recipe page 80) or nut spread
nutmeg, thyme
parsley

Peel and halve potatoes and steam them until softish. Put them on an oven-proof dish with the cut side down. Cover with vegetable broth. Season and roast in the oven until the liquid has thickened. Add cream or nut spread and continue roasting until the potatoes are lightly browned. Serve with the cut facing up and sprinkle with chopped parsley.

Lyonnaise potatoes
1 tbs organic nut spread
½ tbs olive oil

3 small potatoes
1 small onion

Heat organic margarine and oil. Peel potatoes and cut into slices. Cook in liquid fat until softish. Add sliced onion and finish cooking.

Ayurveda potatoes
(An attractive, aromatic dish that yields 3–4 helpings.)
5 large potatoes
½ soy drink
1 package of soy crème (substitute for crème fraîche)
1 bunch each of fresh dill, fresh chives and fresh parsley
juice of ½ lemon
1–2 tsp turmeric
½ tsp curry
soy sauce

Cut the cleaned potatoes into thick slices and cook them for approx. 5 minutes. In the meantime, slowly heat the soy drink in a pan, mixed with the soy crème (do not boil). Stir in turmeric and curry to taste and season with soy sauce. Put the potato slices in the sauce and simmer for approx. 10 minutes. Sprinkle the fresh, finely chopped herbs on the potatoes and serve at once.

Cereal dishes

Japanese rice
80 g wholegrain rice
1½–2 dl vegetable bouillon
1 pinch rock salt
10 g organic nut spread or olive oil
1 small peeled onion studded with clove and bay leaf

Put the rice and studded onion in the bouillon and boil for 40 minutes. Leave to cool and remove the onion. Reheat the rice in the oven and top with heated nut spread or olive oil before serving.

Risotto

80 g wholegrain rice
½ tbs organic nut spread or olive oil
1 tbs chopped onion
2 dl vegetable broth or water
1 pinch rock salt
dried mushrooms
fresh herbs to taste
rosemary
10 g fresh butter* or nut spread
10 g Parmesan cheese* (optional)

Sauté onion in the margarine, add rice and sauté until rice is translucent. Add the vegetable broth or hot water and cook until al dente (30–40 minutes). Add the finely chopped, dried mushrooms and herbs and cook briefly. Before serving, mix in butter, nut spread or olive oil and grated Parmesan cheese with a fork.

Saffron rice

Prepare like risotto. Dissolve a knife tip of saffron powder in a little bouillon and add to rice.

Riz creole with vegetables

½ tbs organic nut spread or olive oil
80 g wholegrain rice
2 tbs finely diced vegetables
(leeks, celery root/celeriac, carrots)
2 dl vegetable broth
1 pinch rock salt
freshly chopped herbs to taste

Briefly sauté rice and vegetables, add hot vegetable broth and herbs, and cook for 30–45 minutes.

Tomato rice

80 g wholegrain rice
½ tbs organic nut spread or olive oil
1 tbs chopped onion
a small amount of garlic, pressed
1 large tomato
approx. 1 dl vegetable broth
1 pinch rock salt
rosemary, marjoram, nutmeg
basil (optional)
a small amount of whole cane sugar
10 g organic nut spread or olive oil

Sauté onion and garlic in nut spread or olive oil, add rice and sauté until the rice is translucent. Add peeled, diced tomato. Add vegetable broth and spices and cook for 30–45 minutes. Add nut spread or olive oil before serving.

Rice with courgettes

½ tbs organic nut spread
80 g wholemeal rice
1 tbs chopped onion
150 g tender courgettes
1 pinch rock salt
1 ½ dl vegetable broth or water
freshly chopped dill
10 g organic nut spread or olive oil

Dice the courgettes. Prepare dish as for tomato rice (see above).

Rice with spinach

80 g wholemeal rice
½ tbs organic nut spread or olive oil
100 g spinach
a small amount of chopped onion
2 dl vegetable broth or water
1 pinch rock salt
nutmeg and peppermint
10 g nut spread

Cut spinach coarsely. Prepare dish as for tomato rice (see above).

Rice with peas (Risi bisi)

80 g wholegrain rice
150 g garden peas, shelled
½ tbs organic nut spread or olive oil
a small amount of chopped onion
1 pinch each fruit sugar and rock salt
½ dl vegetable broth
1 ½–2 dl water
10 g nut spread
parsley

Sauté onion with fruit sugar and a pinch of salt in the margarine. Add the peas and cook briefly, then add vegetable broth and cook the peas until soft. Prepare risotto (according to the recipe on page 95) in a separate pan. Add the peas to the cooked risotto. Before serving, top the prepared rice with nut spread or olive oil and chopped parsley.

Indian rice
80 g wholegrain rice
2 dl vegetable broth
1 pinch rock salt
1 small banana
1 small apple
1 tbs raisins
1 tsp sunflower seeds
1 tsp sesame seeds
saffron, curry, fresh ginger root

Cook rice with vegetable broth and 1 pinch of rock salt until not quite soft (approx. 30–40 minutes). Mix the sliced banana, the peeled and sliced apple, and the raisins into the rice and continue boiling for 5–10 minutes. Season with saffron, curry and grated ginger root to taste. Sprinkle with sunflower seeds and lightly dry-roasted sesame seeds (without fat).

Polenta
½ tbs olive oil
50 g maize semolina, medium fine
3 dl water
nutmeg
1 pinch rock salt
½ tbs nut spread or olive oil

Oil pan. Boil water and stir in the maize. Boil for 5 minutes over low heat, stirring frequently. Season and continue boiling for 45–60 minutes over low heat. Add nut spread or olive oil before serving. You may also add onion slices sautéed without fat.

Millet risotto with vegetables
40 g millet
1 tbs chopped onion
2 tbs finely chopped vegetable cubes (leek, celery root/celeriac, carrots or carrots and peas)
1½ dl vegetable broth
a pinch of rock salt
rosemary
1 tbs grated cheese* (optional)
10 g fresh butter* or nut spread

Sauté onion, diced vegetable and hot-rinsed millet until glazed. Add hot vegetable broth, season and boil for 20 minutes. When serving, add grated cheese* (optional) and a little butter or nut spread flakes or olive oil.

Coarse-ground grain mash
2 tbs coarse-ground grain (wheat, oats, rye)
3 tbs water
1 pinch rock salt

Soak the coarse-ground grain for 12 hours. Then boil in water for 10 minutes or cook for ½ hour in a bain-marie. Add a pinch of salt.

Pasta, spaghetti, macaroni, etc.
For a curative diet, egg pasta should not be used. Today there are high quality wholemeal pastas, soy pastas and spelt pastas in addition to the well-known Italian pasta products made from wheat. There are also many ready-prepared sauces, though these usually contain too much fat (oil, butter, cheese, cream). The most easily digested pasta products are cooked al dente with a classic or simple tomato sauce (see recipes in the chapter 'Sauces').

Spätzle or Knöpfli (without egg)
60 g wholemeal flour
20 g soy flour
1 dl 1:1 diluted milk
1 l water
1 pinch rock salt
1 tbs organic nut spread or olive oil
onion, julienned
chives and parsley

Mix wholemeal and soy flour thoroughly with diluted milk and knead the mixture until the dough forms bubbles. Leave to stand for at least 1 hour.
Boil water with rock salt. Press the dough in portions through a coarse screen into the boiling water or place it on a small wooden cutting board. Cut fine strips with a knife and place them in the boiling water. Let the Knöpfli or Spätzle simmer until they rise to the surface. Take them out with a skimmer and place them on a hot platter. As desired, garnish with julienned onion sautéed in nut spread (or without fat), chives and parsley.

Spinach or tomato Knöpfli*
70 g wholemeal flour ($^1/_3$ soy flour)
1 egg*
1 dl 1:1 diluted milk
1 handful of chopped, raw spinach
or 1 tsp tomato puree
1 dl water
1 pinch rock salt
chives and parsley

Make a smooth batter from the wholemeal and soy flour, egg and water, and leave to stand for 1 hour. Prepare and cook Knöpfli or Spätzle according to the recipe on page 96. Add spinach or tomato puree. Season with chives and parsley.

Oat flake roasts
$^1/_2$ tbs organic nut spread
1 tbs chopped onion
2 tsp of chopped leek, celery, spinach
50 g oat flakes
$^1/_2$ dl vegetable broth
nut spread or olive oil
peppermint or sage

Steam onions and vegetables in nut spread or olive oil, add oat flakes and vegetable broth and cook to a thick mash. Season. Spread approx. 1 cm high on a board and leave to cool. Cut into rectangles. Heat nut spread or olive oil and toast both sides to a golden yellow.

Spinach omelette*
50 g wholemeal flour
1 egg*
100 g 1:1 diluted milk
rock salt
25 g raw, chopped spinach
10 g organic nut spread

Process all ingredients into a smooth dough and leave to stand. Bake omelettes in the heated nut spread.

Sauces

Sauces are a challenge for those on a healing diet, since almost all sauce recipes contain a large amount of fat (butter, oil, cream), cheese and eggs. The combination of hot fat and flour (classic béchamel sauce) should always be avoided. We have put together a few permissible sauces here, whose recipes differ from the classical ones. All of them taste really great.

Béchamel sauce without egg (recipe 1)
For 4 persons:
2–3 tbs wheat flour
1 l milk* or water
1 bay leaf
1 tbs vegetable broth
1 grated onion
1 pinch each rock salt, nutmeg and freshly ground white pepper
chopped parsley

Briefly cook the flour without fat until it is aromatic (it must not turn dark), then let cool slightly. Add the milk or water, bay leaf, vegetable broth and onion while stirring constantly. Bring to the boil. Season. After approx. 5 minutes, remove the bay leaf and serve the sauce sprinkled with parsley.

This basic sauce can be used to make many versions. For example:

Horseradish sauce: When completed, add 10 grammes finely grated horseradish and cook the sauce for another 5 minutes.

Caper sauce: Season the finished sauce with whole or chopped capers and lemon juice.

Olive sauce: Briefly cook the sauce with 4–5 tablespoons tomato puree and 2 tablespoons chopped olives. Season with a knife point of cayenne pepper (optional).

Herb sauce: Add a large quantity of finely chopped herbs such as parsley, lovage, chervil, basil, estragon, oregano, etc. into the finished sauce.

Mushroom sauce: Mix 3–4 tablespoons of very finely chopped raw mushrooms into the finished sauce and season with lemon juice.

Béchamel sauce (recipe 2)
For 4 persons:
2 tbs wheat flour
$1/2$ l soy milk
1 bay leaf
1 onion, finely grated
2 tsp red miso
1 pinch each of pepper and paprika
chopped parsley

Briefly brown the flour without fat until it gives off a toasted aroma. Leave to cool briefly then add the soy milk while stirring constantly. Add the bay leaf and onion and boil for about 5 minutes.
Stir in the miso, remove the bay leaf and season the sauce with pepper and paprika. Sprinkle with chopped parsley.

Miso is a fermented soybean paste that is excellent for seasoning. It tastes like soy sauce but does not contain table salt.

Tomato sauce, classic
$1/2$ tbs organic nut spread or olive oil
1 tbs onion
$1/2$ garlic clove, pressed
2 tbs carrot, celery root/celeriac, leek
2 small tomatoes
1 pinch rock salt
1 pinch whole cane sugar
1 tsp tomato puree
$1 1/2$ dl vegetable broth or water
bay leaf, rosemary, thyme

Sauté the chopped onion, pressed garlic and coarsely cut vegetables in nut spread or olive oil. Add the diced tomatoes and the tomato puree, then add vegetable broth (or water). Season and simmer for $1/2$ hour. Strain if desired.

Tomato sauce, simple
3 tomatoes
1 pinch each rock salt and whole cane sugar
chives, basil
1 tbs olive oil

Dice tomatoes, sauté until soft, season and drain. Add olive oil to taste.

Classic mayonnaise recipe*
For 4 persons:
1 egg yolk*
1 tbs lemon juice
2 dl oil
1 pinch rock salt
onion, herbs

Beat the egg yolk thoroughly with several drops of lemon juice. Add the oil drop by drop while stirring evenly with the whisk. If the mayonnaise becomes too thick, dilute with lemon juice. Season to taste.

Remoulade sauce, classic*
For 4 persons:
Prepare mayonnaise according to above recipe.
1 hardboiled egg*, chopped
1 tbs cornichons, chopped capers
1 tsp parsley, chopped
tomato, diced

Mix the various ingredients with the finished mayonnaise. Garnish with diced tomato.

Mayonnaise without animal protein and fat
See recipe page 82.

Remoulade sauce without animal-based protein
For 4 persons:
Prepare mayonnaise without animal-based protein and fat (see recipe page 82) and mix with 1 tablespoon chopped cornichons, capers and chopped parsley. Garnish with diced tomato.

Vinaigrette*
For 4 persons:
2 tbs olive oil
2 tbs ground nut oil
2 1/2 tbs lemon juice
2 dl water or vegetable broth
1/2 onion, chopped
1 egg*, hardboiled and chopped
1–2 cornichons, cut or finely chopped
parsley or chives
1 tbs tomato, diced
1 pinch rock salt

Whisk oil, lemon juice and vegetable broth until smooth, then add the other ingredients, while mixing thoroughly. The egg is optional.

Sandwiches

Sandwiches are popular as appetizers and summer meals, and to take along on hikes and journeys.
Spreads and ingredients can be used in any number of ways, and various wholemeal types of bread are available, some pre-sliced.
Remember that many loaves are made just to look 'wholemeal' by means of artificial colouring and added grains. Do use real wholemeal bread or pumpernickel.

The recipes are for 4 persons.

Basic spreads
For the strict diet, simply spread organic nut spread on the bread rolls and fill with raw food.

Guacamole (avocado mousse)
2 ripe avocados
juice of 1/2 lemon
1/2 small onion, chopped
2 garlic cloves, pressed
rock salt and white pepper (optional)

Mash the flesh removed from the avocados together with the lemon juice in a blender. Add the onion and garlic and season with rock salt and white pepper. If desired, stir in 1 tablespoon soy cream (instead of crème fraiche).

Sweet avocado cream
1 ripe avocados
4 tbs fresh orange juice
1 tbs honey
1 knife tip ginger powder

Mash the removed pulp of the avocado by squeezing it out or blending it and mix in the other ingredients. Serve at once.

Tofu spread with nuts
250 g tofu, pureed
2 finely chopped spring onions
50 g nuts (hazelnuts, walnuts, almonds, cashew nuts)
rock salt and white pepper (optional)

Lightly roast the nuts in the oven or a dry pan, let cool. Grind the roasted nuts and mix with the pureed tofu and onion. Season with rock salt and pepper.

Quark spread with herbs*
100 g quark
10 g organic nut spread
miso or rock salt

caraway, chives or herbs (dill, borage, lovage, basil, oregano, peppermint etc.)

Stir quark and nut spread to a frothy consistency, season and add individual herbs (or a mix) for variety.

Garnishes
Spreads can be garnished in the following ways:
with raw carrots or celery root/celeriac, with tomatoes, fresh cucumbers, radish, cress, onion rings, nuts, parsley, chives etc.

Desserts

The following recipes are for 4 persons.

Desserts should be eaten with great restraint. Use whole sugar, honey, maple syrup or thickened pear juice for sweetening. Because of their strong flavour, these are not suitable for all recipes, such as vanilla cream. Acacia honey is best for this. If a flavour of its own is to be avoided, moderate amounts of fructose can be used. Agar-agar should be used as a gelling agent. Agar-agar is a vegetable gelatine that is used for vegetable and fruit spreads, sauces and puddings, etc. instead of animal gelatine. All recipes should be made only of organically grown fruits and ingredients. As long as the first two diet stages are needed, sweets should only be eaten on Sundays, at celebrations or with visitors.

Iced soup
50 g whole cane sugar or 80 g acacia honey
4 dl water or
2 dl water or 2 dl grape juice
800 g apricots or peaches or plums, Reineclaude

Boil sugar and liquid together. Briefly cook the pitted, halved fruits in syrup, let cool and prepare beautiful presentation.

Fruit salad
2 tbs acacia honey or 80 g whole cane sugar
1 dl water
1–2 dl organic grape juice or organic apple juice
1–2 tbs lemon juice
600 g apricots or peaches, melons, apples, pears (ripe), red cherries, pitted, berries, grapes

Briefly boil water and honey and let cool. Add grape and lemon juice. Slice seasonal fruits thinly and add to the syrup.

Filled melons
2 small rock melons
Prepare fruit salad according to above recipe.

Halve the melons, scoop out the seeds and fill the melons with the fruit salad.

Fruit jelly
3 dl water or organic grape juice
60 g fruit sugar or 1–2 tbs acacia honey
10 g agar-agar, powdered
7 dl fruit juice from oranges, berries

Mix water well with fructose or honey and agar-agar and heat over a low heat. Stir frequently until the agar-agar has completely dissolved. Add fruit juice and serve immediately in glasses or desert cups. Garnish with sesame cream to taste (see recipe page 80).

Apple puree
800 g apples
2 dl water or organic apple juice
1–2 tbs acacia honey
cinnamon or 1 grated lemon peel (from untreated lemons)

Remove stem and calyx from the apples, cut the apples into pieces, cook them with the water or fruit juice until soft, and mix well. Add honey and cinnamon or lemon peel (organic lemons). If you like, you can add almond paste. From the third diet level onwards, soy cream may be used as garnish.

Apple or pear compote
800 g apples or pears
2–3 dl water or organic apple juice
1 tbs acacia honey
1 grated lemon peel (from untreated lemons) or cinnamon

Core and peel the apples or pears, and cut them into wedges. Bring water or juice to a boil, add honey and lemon peel or cinnamon, add the fruit, and cook until soft.

Baked apples (recipe 1)
800 g apples
½ dl water or organic apple juice
1 tbs honey
¼ cinnamon stick
quince, raspberry or currant jelly (see recipe page 100) or raisins and wine berries with a touch of honey

Boil water or apple juice with honey and cinnamon stick. Peel, core, halve and place apple portions in the hot water or juice. Cook slowly until soft. Remove with skimmer and place on a flat platter with the cut surface up. Fill the apples with jelly or mix of raisin, wine, berry and honey.

Baked apples (recipe 2)
4 large or 8 small apples
4 tbs currants
4 tbs sesame cream (see recipe page 80)
1–2 tbs honey
grated lemon peel (untreated lemon)
10 g nut spread or almond spread
1 tbs maple syrup
1–2 dl organic apple juice

Mix hazelnuts, currants, sesame cream, honey and lemon peel, fill the prepared apples (cored and peeled) and place the apples in a casserole. Add nut spread or maple syrup and pour 1 cm apple juice over the apples. Bake for 20–30 min.

Dried fruit salad with grapes and pine nuts
200 g dried figs
200 g dates
200 g dried apples
400 g grapes
juice of 1 lemon
2 tbs honey
50 g pine nuts

Chop the dried fruit, halve one half of the grapes and squeeze the others. Put all fruits in a dish. Mix the lemon juice and grape juice with the honey and pour it over the fruits. Cool before serving. Toast the pine nuts and sprinkle them over the fruit salad.

Strawberry or raspberry cream
300 g berries
vanilla cream
1–2 dl sesame cream (see recipe page 80)

Prepare a vanilla cream according to the recipe on page 102 and mix with the mixed or pureed berries. Fold in sesame cream or serve separately.

Lemon cream
¼ l organic whole milk
1–2 lemons, untreated
1 tbs cornflour or arrowroot flour
3 tbs whole milk
2 tbs acacia honey
sesame cream (see recipe page 80) to taste

Slice lemon peel thin and boil in the milk. Add cornflour or arrowroot flour stirred with a little cold milk and boil briefly. Add honey and return to the pan, stirring constantly, and heat almost to the boil. Strain the cooled cream and add a few spoons of lemon juice and sesame cream to taste.

Orange cream
Prepare as lemon cream (see recipe page 101).

Orange aspics
5 dl fresh orange juice
5 g agar-agar, powdered
(= vegetable jelly)
1 tbs fruit sugar

Mix thoroughly 3 dl orange juice, agar-agar and sugar and heat over a low flame while stirring constantly (do not boil) until the agar-agar has dissolved completely. Add the remaining orange juice and pour it into chilled moulds. Keep cold.

Sesame bars
100 g Syramena sugar
2 tbs honey
100 g sesame seeds, whole not ground

Syramena sugar is a light raw cane sugar available in health-food stores. Heat the sugar in a dry pan and stir until a light caramel forms. Add the liquid honey and mix well. Add the sesame and mix well again. Pour the mass into a mould or onto an oiled board, let cool slightly and cut into squares or diamonds. Let cool.

Vanilla cream
1 vanilla pod
¼ l water
40 g wheat flour (white flour as an exception)
3 tbs honey
approx. 200 ml soy milk

Cut into the vanilla bean with a sharp knife, scrape out the pulp and place everything in the water to boil. Put the wheat flour into the vanilla water while stirring constantly and let it swell into a thick mash. Let it cool slightly, then stir in the honey and soy milk. Depending on the amount of soy milk, you will get vanilla cream or vanilla sauce. Keep cool until serving.

Vanilla sauce
See vanilla cream (see recipe page 102)

Almond milk sauce
4 dl organic whole milk
50 g almonds or almond spread
2 tbs honey
1 tbs cornflour or arrowroot flour
2 tbs water

Boil milk with the peeled, ground almonds (or the almond spread) and honey. Stir cornflour or arrowroot flour in cold water and stir into the boiling milk. Mix the finished sauce.

Rosehip sauce
70 g rosehip puree or rosehip pulp
2 dl water or grape juice
1–2 tbs honey
a few drops of lemon juice (optional)

Boil the ingredients together, then add the lemon juice.

Red wine sauce
2 dl water
lemon or orange peel (untreated fruits)
1 cinnamon stalk
1 clove
1–2 tbs acacia honey
2 dl red grape juice, organic
20 g almonds

Boil water, peel, spices and honey together for a few minutes, then strain. Add grape juice and heat (do not boil). Add peeled and sliced almonds.

Red fruit jelly (chilled soup)
7 dl currant, raspberry or strawberry juice
3 dl red grape juice or water
70 g semolina
1 tbs maize flour

Boil berry juice and grape juice together, stir in semolina and cornflour and boil for 10 minutes. Pour into rinsed pudding mould and store in cool place. Serve with vanilla sauce (see recipe page 102) or almond milk sauce (see recipe page 102).

Red fruit jelly, Danish style
1 kg berries (raspberries, currants, strawberries or pitted cherries, or all mixed)
½ l fruit juice (e.g. elderberry)
2 packs of agar-agar
honey to taste
½ teaspoon natural vanilla
sesame cream, liquid (see recipe page 80)

Put cleaned and chopped (optional) fruits into a dish, mix with honey and vanilla. Heat the fruit juice with agar-agar and pour the liquid over the fruits. Let the fruit jelly harden. Serve with liquid sesame cream.

Blueberry mash (Heitisturm)
1 kg blueberries
160 g whole cane sugar
2 dl water
1 tbs organic wholemeal flour
2 tbs water
2 tbs olive oil
20 g wholemeal bread cubes

Cook the blueberries with sugar and water for 5 minutes, stir wholemeal flour into water, add to blueberry mixture, boil briefly and prepare the mash. Add the pieces of bread roasted in olive oil.

Rhubarb compote
1 kg rhubarb
120–160 g whole cane sugar
1 dl water
½ tbs maize or arrowroot flour (optional)

Peel the rhubarb and, if necessary, dice. Add sugar and water and cook briefly until soft. Take out the rhubarb pieces with a skimmer and arrange them. Cook the juice briefly, reduce slightly with maize meal and arrange on the compote.

Strawberry coupe
500 g strawberries
80 g fruit sugar
1 tbs heaped almond puree or soy cream (recipe see page 80)

Mix the berries. Add sugar and slowly mix with almond puree or soy cream. Garnish with whole berries.
This recipe can be prepared with many other fruits.

Fruit coupe
250 g fruits (pears, apricots, peaches, berries)
2 dl water
2–3 tbs fruit sugar
2 tbs almond puree

Cut the fruits into pieces and mix them finely with the almond puree. Garnish with beaten soy cream.

Apple cream
400 g apples
¼ litre of freshly prepared almond milk
½ vanilla bean
1 tbs maize flour or arrowroot flour
1 tbs whole milk
1 tbs fruit sugar
½ dl water or organic apple juice
1 ground organic lemon peel
1 tbs heaped almond puree

Prepare a thick apple sauce (for the recipe, see page 100) and mix with almond puree.

Recipes

Almond milk	79
Almond milk sauce	102
Almond puree dressing	82
Apple compote	101
Apple creme	103
Apple muesli	77
Apple puree	100
Apples, baked (recipe 1)	101
Apples, baked (recipe 2)	101
Artichokes	91
Asparagus	91
Aubergines	91
Baked fennel with cream cheese sauce	88
Basic spreads for sandwiches	
– Basic spread	99
– Guacamole (avocado mousse)	99
Bircher muesli	77
Blueberry mash (Heitisturm)	103
Broccoli	91
Broccoli soup	87
Cabbage or white cabbage, steamed	91
Carrots, cooked	89
Carrot soup	87
Cauliflower	91
Cauliflower soup	87
Celery root/celeriac, steamed	89
Celery stalks	88
Cereal dishes	94
Chervil soup	87
Chicory/endive, sautéed	88
Chilled soup	79
Cleaning leafy vegetables	81
Coarse-ground grain mash	96
Cooked food	84
Courgettes with tomatoes	90
Cream dressing	82

Desserts	100
Dried fruit salad with grapes and pine nuts	101
Filled melons	100
Fresh grain cereal mash	78
Fruit and fresh grain dishes	78
Fruit coupe	103
Fruit jelly	100
Fruit juices	76
Fruit salad	100
Garnishes	100
Green beans with tomatoes	89
Gruel to accompany juices	77
Iced soup	100
Juices	76
Knöpfli, without egg	96
Lemon cream	101
Lettuce	88
Macaroni	96
Mayonnaise, classic recipe	82
Mayonnaise, vegan	82
Milk types (vegetable milk)	79
Millet risotto with vegetables	96
Minestrone	87
Mixed – pureed raw vegetables	83
Oat cream soup	86
Oat flake roasts	97
Oat groat soup	86
Oil dressing (mild)	81
Orange aspics	102
Orange cream	102

Pasta	96
Pasta, wholemeal	96
Pear compote	101
Peas and carrots	89
Pine nut milk	80
Polenta	96
Potato dishes	93
– Ayurveda potatoes	94
– Baked potato	93
– Bouillon potatoes	93
– Caraway potatoes	93
– Lyonnaise potatoes	94
– Mashed potatoes	94
– Potatoes in their skin	93
– Potatoes with tomatoes	93
– Roast potatoes	94
Potato juice	77
Potato salad	92
Potato salad with cucumbers	92
Potato soup	87
Pureed raw vegetables	83
Quark dressing	81
Quark spread with herbs	99
Raspberry cream	101
Ratatouille	90
Raw vegetables and salads	80
Raw vegetables, mixed	82
Red cabbage	92
Red fruit jelly (chilled soup)	102
Red fruit jelly, Danish style	103
Rhubarb compote	103
Rice dishes	
– Indian rice	96
– Japanese rice	94
– Rice with courgettes	95
– Rice with peas	95
– Rice with spinach	95
– Risi bisi	95
– Risotto	95
– Riz creole with vegetables	95
– Saffron rice	95
– Tomato rice	95
Rice soup, clear	85
Rice soup, thickened	86

Salad dressings	81
Salad dressing table	83
Salade niçoise	92
Salads and raw vegetables	80
Salads of cooked vegetables	92
Sandwiches	99
Sauces	97
– Béchamel sauce without egg (recipe 1)	97
– Béchamel sauce (recipe 2)	98
– Caper sauce	98
– Herb sauce	98
– Horseradish sauce	97
– Mayonnaise, classic	98
– Mushroom sauce	98
– Olive sauce	98
– Red wine sauce	102
– Remoulade, classic	98
– Remoulade sauce without animal-based protein	99
– Rosehip sauce	102
– Tomato sauce, classic	98
– Tomato sauce, simple	98
– Vinaigrette	99
Sauerkraut salad	83
Semolina dumplings	85
Sesame bars	102
Sesame cream	80
Sesame frappé	80
Sesame milk	80
Sesame puree dressing	82
Snow peas, cooked	89
Soups	85
Soy milk	80
Spaghetti	96
Spätzle, without egg	96
Spinach, chopped	88
Spinach Knöpfli	97
Spinach omelette	97
Spinach soup	87
Spinach, whole leaves	88
Sprouted cereal grains	79
Strawberry coupe	103
Strawberry cream	101
Sugar peas, cooked	89
Summer tomato soup	86
Sweet avocado cream	99
Sweet peppers (green, yellow, red)	90

Table of salad dressings	83	Vegetable broth	85
Tofu spread with nuts	99	Vegetable curry	89
Tomatoes à la Provençale	90	Vegetable juices	76
Tomatoes, baked	90	Vegetables	88
Tomatoes, raw, stuffed	83	Vegetables,	
Tomatoes, stewed	90	mixed – pureed raw	83
Tomato Knöpfli	97	Vegetable soups, various	87
Tomato soup	86		
		White cabbage or	
Vanilla cream	102	cabbage, steamed	91
Vanilla sauce	102		
Vegetable aspics	93	Yoghurt dressing	81
Vegetable bouillon	85		

Notes

1 Endepols, H. et al., *'Effort based decision making in the rat: a (18F) fluodeoxiglucose micro positron emitting tomography study'*, J Neurosci 20 (29) 2010, 7908–14.
2 Di Paolo et al., *'Chronic exposure to aluminium and melatonin through the diet: neurobehavioral effects in a transgenig mous model of Alzheimer disease*, Food Chem toxicol. 2014 July, 69, 320–29.
3 Huppelsberg, J. et al.: *Kurzlehrbuch der Physiologie*, 4th ed. Thieme-Verlag, 223.
4 Ransohoff, R.M. et al., *'The myeloid cells of the central nervous system parenchyma'*, Nature 468, no. 7312, 2010, 253–62, PMID 21068834.
5 Fagerholm, U., *'The highly permeable blood-brain barrier: an evaluation of current pinions about brain uptake capacity'*, Drug discovery today 12, 2007, 1076–82, PMID 18061888 (review).
6 Chiu, W.L. et al., *'Linear correlation of the fraction of oral dose absorbed of 64 drugs between humans and rats'*, Pharm Res 15, 1998, 1792–95, PMID 9834005.
7 Goodwin, U.T. et al., *'In silico predictions of blood-brain barrier penetration: considerations to 'keep in mind''*, J pharmacol Exp ther 315, 2005, 477–83, PMID 15919767 (review).
8 Mato, M. et al., *'Evidence for the possible function of the fluorescent granular perithelial cells in brain as scavengers of high-molecular marker ED-2'*, Experientia 40, 1984, 399–402, PMID 6325229.
9 Balabanov, R. et al., *'CNS vascular pericytes express macrophage-like function, cell-surface integrin alpha M, a macrophage marker ED-2'*, Microvasc Res 52, 1996, 127–42, PMID 8901442.
10 Hickey, W.F. et al., *'Perivascular microglial cells of the CNS are bone-marrow derived and present antigen in vivo'*, Science 239, 1988, 290–92, PMID 3276004.
11 Fabry, Z. et al., *'Differential activation of Th1 und Th2 CD4+ cells by murine brain microvessel endothelial cells and smooth muscle pericytes'*, J Immunol 151, 1993, 38–47, PMID 8100844.
12 Täuble, H., *'Carriers and specificity in membranes. E. Carrier-facilitates transport. Kinks as carriers in membranes'*, Neurosci Res Program Bull 9, 1971, 361–372, PMID 5164654.
13 Träuble, H., *'Phasenumwandlungen in Lipiden. Mögliche Schaltprozesse in biologischen Membranen'*, Naturwissenschaften 58, 1971, 277–284, PMID 4935358 (review).
14 Vastowsky, O., *'Chemie der Naturstoffe-Lipoproteine und Membranen'* (http://www.chemie.uni erlangen.de/0c/vostrowsky/naturstoff/03 Membranen. pdf), Universität Erlangen, 2005, 42.
15 Timai, I. et al., *'Structure internalization relationship for adsorptive mediated endocytosis of basic peptides at the blood-brain barrier'*, J Pharmacol Exp Ther 280, 1997, 10–15, ONUD 8996222.
16 Weiss, N. et al., *'The blood-brain barrier in brain homeostasis and neurological diseases'*, Biochem. Biophys. Acta 1788, 2009, 842–57 (review).
17 Banks, W.A. et al., *'Cytokines and the blood-brain-barrier'*, Siegel, A. et al., *'The neuroimmunological basis of behavior and mental disorders'*, Springer, New York, 2009, 3–17.
18 Hill, H.U., *'Umweltschadstoffe und neurodegenerative Erkrankungen des Gehirns'*, Demenzkrankheiten, Shaker-Verlag Aachen 2010, 62–63.
19 Comford, E.M. et al., *'Comparison of lipid-mediated blood-brain-barrier permeability in neonates and adults'* Am J Physiol-Cell Physiol 243, 1982, 161C–68C, PMID 7114247.
20 Elmas, I. et al., *'Effects of profound hypothermia on the blood-brain-barrier in brain homeostasis and neurological diseases'*, Forensic Science International 119, 2001, 212–16, PMID 11376985.
21 Phillips, S.C. et al., *'Weakening of the blood-brain-barrier by alcohol-related stresses in the rat'*, J Neurol Sci 54, 1982, 271–78, PMID 7201507.
22 Sing, A.K. et al., *'Effects of chronic alcohol drinking on the blood brain barrier and ensuing neuronal*

toxicity in alcohol-preferring rats subjected to intraperitoneal LPS injection, *J Neurol Sci* 54, 1982, 271–78, PMID 7201507.
23. Haorah, J. et al., *'Alcohol-induced blood-brain-barrier dysfunction is mediated via inositol 1,4,5-triphosphate receptor (IP3R)-gated intracellular calcium release'*, *J Neurochem* 100, 2007, 324–336, PMID 1724115.
24. Haorah, J. et al., *'Ethanol-induced activation of myosin light chain kinase leads to dysfunction of tight junctions and blood-brain-barrier compromise. Alcoholism'*, *Clinical and Experimental Research* 29, 2005, 999–1009, PMID 15976526.
25. Haorah, J. et al., *'Alcohol induced oxidative stress in brain endothelial cells causes blood-brain-barrier dysfunction'*, *J of Leukocye Biology* 78, 2005, 1223–32, PMID 16204625.
26. Peters, R. et al., *'Smoking, dementia and cognitive decline in the elderly, a systematic review'*, *BMC Geriatr* 8, 2008, 36, PMID 19105840 (review).
27. Lockman, P.R. et al., *'Brain uptake kinetics of nicotine and cotinine after chronic nicotine exposure'*, *J Pharmacol Exp Ther* 314, 2005, 636–642, PMID 15845856.
28. Chen, Y.H. et al., *'Enhanced Escherichia coli invasion of human brain microvascular endothelial cells is associated with alternations in cytoskeleton induced by nicotine'*, *Cell Microbiol* 4, 2002, 503–14, PMID 12174085.
29. D'Andrea, D.A. et al., *'Microwave effects on the nervous system'*, *Bioelectromagnetics* 6, 2003, 107–174, PMID 14628310 (review).
30. Patel, T.H. et al., *'Blood-brain-barrier dysfunction associated with increased expression of tissue and urokinase plasminogen activators following peripheral thermal injury'*, *Neurosci Lett* 444, 2008, 222–26, PMID 18719505.
31. Salford, L.G. et al., *'Nerve cell damage in mammalian brain after exposure to microwaves from GSM mobile phones'*, *Environ Health Perspect* 111, 2003, 881–883, PMID 12782486.
32. Nittby, H. et al., *'Radiofrequency and extremely low-frequency electromagnetic field effects on the blood-brain-barrier'*, *Electromagn Biol Med* 27, 2008, 215–229, PMID 18821198.
33. Eberhardt, J.L. et al., *'Blood-brain-barrier permeability and nerve cell damage in rat brain 14 and 28 days after exposure to microwaves from GSM mobile phones'*, *Electromagn Biol Med* 27, 2008, 215–229, PMID 18821198.
34. Salford, L.G. et al., *'Permeability of the blood-brain-barrier induced by 914 MHz electromagnetic radiation, continuous wave and modulated at 8, 16, 50 and 200 Hz'*, *Microsc Res Tech* 2727, 1994, 245–542, PMID 8012056.
35. Meyl, K., *'Elektromagnetische Umweltverträglichkeit'*, Umdruck zum Informationstechnischen Seminar, Indel GmbH Verlagsabteilung Villingen-Schwenningen, 2002, 3rd ed., 81–83.
36. Patel, J.R. et al., *'Moderators of Oligodendrocyte differentiation during remyelinisation'*, doi:10.1016/j.febslet.2011.04.037.
37. Shen, S. et al., *'Age-dependent epigenetic control of differentiation inhibitors is critical for remyelinisation efficiency'*, *Nature Neurosciensce* 11 (9), 1024–34.
38. Hanafy, K.H. et al., *'Regulation of Remyelinisation in multiple sclerosis'*, *FEBS-letters* 585 (23), 3821–3828.
39. Franklin, R.J.M. et al., *'Remyelinisation in the CNS: from biology to therapy'*, *Nature Reviews Neuroscience* 9 (11), 839–55.
40. Merlini, G. et al., *'Molecular mechanisms of amyloidosis'*, *N Engl J Med* no. 349, 2003, 583–96.
41. Van Wijk, R. et al., Utrecht University: *'An introduction to Human Biophoton Emission'*, *Forsch Komplementärmed Klass Naturheilk.* 2005, 12, 77–83.
42. Gurwitsch, A.G., *Das Problem der Zellteilung*, Springer-Verlag, Berlin, 1926; *Die mitogenetische Zellstrahlung,* Springer-Verlag, Berlin, 1932; Ferner; *Arch R. mikr. Anat. Und Entwicklungsmech,* vols. 51, 52, 100, 101 and 104.
43. Bischof, M, *Biophotonen, das Licht in unseren Zellen,* ISBN 3-86150 095 7.
44. Popp, F.A., *Biologie des Lichtes, Grundlagen der ultraschwachen Zellstrahlung,* Verlag Paul Parex, ISBN: 3-489-61734-7.
45. Rubik, Beverly, *'Natural light from organisms: life at the edge of sciences,'* in Fischer, H., *'Photons as transmitters for intra- and extracellular biological and biochemical communication: the construction of a hypothesis, Electromagnetic Bio-Information,* Popp, F.A., ed., Urban und Schwarzenberg, Munich, 1989, 70.
46. Bircher-Benner M.O., *Grundzüge der Ernährungstherapie auf Grund der Energie-Spannung*

der Nahrung, Verlag Otto Salle, Berlin, 1905 and 1906.
47 Bircher-Benner, M.O., *'Der zweite Hauptsatz der Energetik und die Ernährung. Zschr der Wendepunkt, Wendepunkt-Verlag, Zürich, 1936 und Vom Wesen und der Organisation der Nahrungsenergie und über die Anwendung des zweiten Hauptsatzes der Energielehre auf den Nährwert und die Nahrungswirkung'*, Kleine Hippokrates-Bücherei, vol. 8, Hippokrates-Verlag Stuttgart and Leipzig 1936.
48 Popp, F.A., *Unsere Lebensmittel in neuer Sicht*, ISBN 3-596-11459-4.
49 Prigogine, I. et al., *Dialog mit der Natur*, Piper-Verlag München, ISBN 3-492-11181-5.
50 Kasnaceev, C.P. in Jezowska-Trzebiatoveska, B. et al., *'Photon emission from biological systems'*, proceedings of the first international symposium, Wroclav Pland Jan, 1986.
51 Harman, D., *'Aging: a theory based on free radical and radication chemistry'* J of Gerontology 11, 1956, 298–300, PMID 13332224.
52 Harman, D., *'The free radical theory of aging'*, Antioxid Redox Signal 5, 2003, 557–561, PMID 14580310.
53 Bockman, K.B. et al., *'Mitochondrial aging: open questions'*, Ann N.Y. Acad Sci 854, 1998, 118–127, PMID 9928425.
54 Sohr Ch., *'Oxydativer Stress bei diabetischer Neuropathie'*, Medizinische Fakultät, Deutsches Diabetes-Zentrum DDZ 2007 (online).
55 Berg, D. et al., *'Parkinson's disease'*, Lajita, A. et al. in *Handbook of Neurochemistry and Molecular Neurology*, 3rd ed., *Degenerative Diseases of the Nervous System*, Springer-Verlag, Berlin, Heidelberg, 2007, 9 ff.
56 Kilburn, K.H., *'Neurobehavioral and pulmonary impairment in 105 adults with indoor exposure to molds compared to 100 exposed to chemicals'*, Toxicol. Ind. Health 25 (9–10) 681–92.
57 Hill, H.U., *Umweltschadstoffe und Neurodegenerative Erkrankungen des Gehirns, Demenzkrankheiten*, Shakefr-Verlag Aachen, 2010, 5.
58 Schäfer, S.G. et al., *Metalle, Lehrbuch der Toxikologie*, Wiss. Verlagsgesellschaft mbH Stuttgart, 2nd ed. 2003, 273 ff.
59 Birkmeyer, J.D.D. et al., *'Quecksilberdepots im Organismus korrelieren mit der Anzahl der Amalgamfüllungen'*, Deutsche Zeitschr für Biologische Zahnmedizin 6, 57–61.

60 Mutter, J. et al., *'Amalgam-Risiko für die Menschheit. Quecksilbervergiftungen richtig ausleiten'*. Fit fürs Leben-Verlag, 2nd ed., Natura Viva Verlags-GmbH, Weil der Stadt, 2006.
61 Drasch, G. et al., *'Mercury burden of human fetal and infant tissues'*, Eur.J. Paediat 1994 (8), 607–10.
62 Olivieri, G. et al., *'The effects of β-estradiol on SHSY6Y neuroblastome cells during heavy metal induced oxidative stress, neurotoxicity and β-Amyloid secretion'*, Neuroci. 113, 849–55.
63 Griem, P. et al., *'Metal-induced autoimmunity'*, Curr Opin Immunol 7 831–39.
64 Grandjean, P. et al., *'Cognitive deficit in seven-year-old children with prenatal exposure to methylmercury'*, Neurotox Toxicol 19, 417–28, 1997.
65 Dott et al., *Lehrbuch der Umweltmedizin*, Wiss. Verlagsgesellschaft Stuttgart 2002, 170 ff.
66 Curth, A., *'Der Einfluss von Quecksilber auf die Entstehung der Alzheimer-Erkrankung: eine systematische Review'*, medical dissertation, Universitätsklinik Freiburg i.B., 2008, http//www.freidoc.uni-freiburg.de/volltexte/6091.
67 Mutter, J. et al., *'Quecksilber und Alzheimer Krankheit'*, Fortschr Neurol Psychiatr 75, 528–38.
68 Greenpeace: dpa Meldung 2000.
69 Schäfer, S.G. et al., *Lehrbuch der Toxikologie*, Wiss. Verlagsgesellschaft mbH. Stuttgart. 2nd ed., 2003, 763 ff.
70 Hill H.U., *Umweltschadstoffe und Neurodegenerative Erkrankungen des Gehirns, Demenzerkrankungen*, Shaker-Verlag, Aachen, 2nd ed.
71 Haga, S. et al., *'Neuronal degeneration and glia-cell responses following trimethylin intoxication in the rat'*, Acta Neuropathol 103 (6), 575–82.
72 Binz, P., *Zehn Fallberichte (Kasuistiken) von Patienten mit Chemikalienbelastung (Organophosphatpestizide, Reinigungsmittel mit Chlorgehalt) aus der neurologischen Praxis*, in Hill, H.U., *Umweltschadstoffe und Neurodegenerative Erkrankungen des Gehirns, Demenzkrankheiten*, Shaker-Verlag Aachen, 2010, 17.
73 Axelson, O. et al., *'A case-referent study on neuropsychiatric disorders among workers exposed to solvents'*, Scand J Work Environ Health 2 14–20.
74 Husmann, K., *'Symptoms of car painters with long-term exposure to organic solvents'*, Scand J Work Environ Health 6, 19–26.
75 Schwartz, E., *'Proportionate mortality ration analysis of automobile mechanics and gasoline service*

station workers in New Hampshire', Am J Ind Med 12, 91–99.

76 Ashford, N.A. et al., 'Chemical exposures: low levels and high stakes', Toxicol Ind Health 3, 1–7.

77 Merz, T. et al., 'Merkblatt zur Bewertung von VOC-Gemischen', Umwelt-Medizin-Gesellschaft 18/4, 2005, 291–93.

78 UBA, 'Richtwerte für Innenraumluft, in Eikmann et al., Gefährdung. Toxikologische Basisdaten und ihre Bewertung, Erich Schmidt-Verlag, Berlin, 2002.

79 Binz, P., Zehn Fallberichte (Kasuistiken) von Patienten mit Chemikalienbelastungen (Organophosphatpestizide, Reinigungsmittel mit Chlorgehalt) aus der neurologischen Praxis, in Hill, H.U., Umweltschadstoffe und Neurodegenerative Erkrankungen des Gehirns, Demenzkrankheiten, Shaker-Verlag, Aachen, 2010, 23–24.

80 Hörr, B., 'Positronen-Emissions-Tomographie (PET)-Befunde von 2 Patienten mit Organophosphat-Pestizid Belastung', in Hill, H.U., 'Umweltschadstoffe und neurodegenerative Erkrankungen des Gehirns, Demenzkrankheiten', Shaker-Verlag, Aachen, 2010, 23–24.

81 Sayal et al., 'Prenatal alcohol exposure and gender differences in children mental health problems: longitudinal population-based study', in Pediatrics 119 (2) 2002. 426–34.

82 Crellin, R. et al., 'Folates and psychiatric disorders, Clinic potential', Drugs 45 1993 (45) 623–36.

83 Herrmann, W., Mitochondriale Medizin Teil 12, 'Homocystein und Neurodegeneration', online article in www.ganzimmun.de, 31 May 2010 (online seminar archive).

84 Durk, M.R. et al., '1α,25-Dihydroxyvitamin D3 reduces cerebral amyloid-β-accumulation and improves cognition in mouse models of Alzheimer's disease', J Neuropsy 2014 May 21, 34 (21), 7091–101.

85 Groves, N.J. et al., 'Vitamin D as a neurosteroid affecting the developing and adult brain', Annu Rev Nutr 2014, 34, 117–41.

86 Kfoszynnska, M. et al., 'The role of vitamin D in multiple sclerosis', Postepy Hit Med Dosw (online) 8 April 2015, 69, 440–6.

87 Schwarz, S. et al., 'Diet and multiple sclerosis', Nervenarzt 2005 Feb 76, 2, 131–42.

88 Boustani, M. et al., 'Screening for Dementia in Primary Care: A Summary of the Evidence for the U.S. Preventive Services Task Force', in Annals of Internal Medicine, vol. 138, no. 11, 3 June 2003, ISSN: 0003-4819 S. 927–37, PMID: 12779304.

89 Alzheimer Report, Kings College, London, 'Alle 3,2 Sekunden erkrankt ein Mensch an Demenz', in focus.de, downloaded 26 August 2015, http//www.focus.de/gesundheit/news/alzheimer-bericht, id 4902927.html).

90 Brinks, R. et al., 'Age- and time-dependent model of the prevalence of non-communicable diseases and application to dementia in Germany', in Theoretical Population Biology, March 2014, PMID 24333220.

91 Nehls, M., Die Alzheimer Lüge. Die Wahrheit über eine vermeidbare Krankheit, Heyne, 2014, ISBN 978-3-453-20069-2.

92 Middleton, M.E. et al., 'Promising strategies for the prevention of dementia', in Arch. Neurol., vol. 66, no. 10, 2009, 2010–15, PMID19822776.

93 Kirshner, H.S., 'Vascular dementia: a review of recent evidence for prevention and treatment', in Neurosci Rep., vol. 9, no. 6, 2009, 437–42, PMID 19818230.

94 Flicker, L., 'Life style interventions to reduce the risk of dementia', in Maturitas 63 (Epub ahead of print), no. 4, 2009, 319–22, PMID 19631480.

95 Korczyn, A.D. et al., 'Is dementia preventable?', in Dialogues Clin Neurosci. 11 (2) 2009, 213–16, PMID 19585956.

96 Alonso, A. et al., 'Cardiovascular risk factors and dementia mortality: 40 years of follow-up in the Seven Countries Study', in J Neurol Sci 280 (Epub), no. 1–2, 2009, 79–83, PMID 19251275.

97 Elwood, P. et al., 'Healthy Lifestyle Reduce the Incidence of Chronic Diseases and Dementia: Evidence from the Caerphilly Cohort Study', in PLOS ONE 8, 2013, e81877, doi:10.1371/journal, Pone.0081877.

98 Yamamoto, T. et al., 'Association between self-reported dental health status and onset of dementia: a 4-year prospective cohort study of older Japanese adults from the Aichi Gerontological Evaluation Study (AGES) Project', in Psychosom. Med. Band 74 (3), 2012, 241–48, PMID 22408130.

99 Mirakhur, A. et al., 'Behavioural and psychological syndromes in Alzheimer's disease', Int J Geriatr Psychiatry, 2004, Nov 19 (11), 1035.39.

100 Rohr, Helga, a.com (http://www.helgarohra.com), downloaded 13 December 2015.

101 European Working Group of People with Dementia, *'Who we are'*, *Alzheimer-europe.de* (http://www.alzheimer-europe.org/Alzheimer-Europe/Who-we-are/European-Working-Group-of-People-with-Dementia), downloaded 13 December 2015.
102 Jessen, F. et al., *'Prediction of Dementia by Subjective Memory Impairment'*, in *Arch Gen Psychiatry* 2010, 67, 414–22.
103 Jessen, F. et al., *'Prediction of dementia in Primary Care Patients'*, in *PLOS ONE*, Research Article, 8 February 2011, doi:10.1371/journal.pone.0016852.
104 Ferri, C. P. et al., *'Global prevalence of dementia: a Delphi consensus study'*, in *Lancet*, vol. 366, no. 3503, Dec 2005, 2112–117, PMID: 16360788.
105 Engel, S., *Alzheimer und Demenzen, Unterstützung für Angehörige*, Trias-Verlag, Stuttgart, 2012, ISBN 9783-8304-3983-7.
106 Alzheimer, A., 'Über eine eigentümliche Krankheit der Hirnrinde', in *Allg. Zeitschr. f. Psychiat.- Psychiat. Gerichtl. Medizin*, 64, 1–2, 1907, 146–48.
107 Script of broadcast *Quarks & Co Zum Thema Alzheimer* (http://www.wdr.de/tv/quarks/global/pdf/gedaechtnis.pdf) (PDF, 612 kB).
108 Emmerich, J., *'Viele scheuen bei Demenz den Gang zum Arzt'*, in derwesten.de, 20 Sept 2010, downloaded 27 Dec 2014, http://www.derwesten.de/nachrichten/Viele-scheuen-bei-demenz-den-Gang-zum-Arzt-id3738233.html).
109 Brookmeyer, R. et al., *'Forecasting the global burden of Alzheimer's disease'*, in *Alzheimers & dementia: journ. of Alzheimer's Assoc.*, vol. 3, no. 3, July 2007, 186–191, PMID 19595937.
110 Jonsson, T. et al., *'A mutation in APP protects against Alzheimer's disease and age related cognitive decline'*, *Nature*, vol. 488, no. 7409, Aug 2012, 96–99, PMID 22801501.
111 Rogaeva, E. et al., *'The neuronal sortilin-related receptor SORL 1 is genetically associated with Alzheimer's disease'*, in *Nature Genetics*, vol. 39, no. 2 Feb 2007, 168–177, PMID 17220890.
112 PSE1 E280A (PAISA) (http://www.alzforum.org/mutation/psen 1 -e280a-paisa), in Alzforum.org, downloaded 27 July 2015.
113 Soscia, S. J. et al., *'The Alzheimer's disease-associated amyloid beta-protein is an antimicrobial peptide'*, in *PLOS one*, vol. 5, no. 3, 2010, e9505, PMID 20209079.

114 Michyo, I. et al., *'Synthetic tau-fibrils mediate transmission of neurofibrillary tangles in a transgenic mouse-model of Alzheimer's like tauopathy'*, *J. Neuroscience*, no. 33, 16 Jan 2013, 1024–37.
115 Mayeux, R. et al., *'Genetic susceptibility and head injury as risk factors for Alzheimer's disease among community-dwelling elderly persons and their first-degree relatives'*, *Ann.neurol.* 33, (5), 1993, 494–501, PMID 8498827.
116 Neumann, K. F. et al., *'Insulin resistance and Alzheimer's disease: molecular links & clinical implications'*, *Curr Alzheimer Res*, no. 5 (5), Oct 2008, 438–447, PMID 18855585.
117 Rohriz-Filho, S. et al., *'(Pre)-diabetes, brain aging, and cognition'*, *Biochem Biophys Acta*, 2009, 432–443, PMID 19135149.
118 Qiu, W. O. et al., *'Insulin, insulin-degrading enzyme and amyloid beta peptide in Alzheimer's disease, review and hypothesis'*, *Neurobiol. Aging*, Feb, 27 (2) 2006, 190–98, PMID 19135149.
119 Kofman, O. S. et al., *'Diffuse cerebral atrophy'*, *Applied therapeutics*, vol. 12 (4), April 1970, 24–26, PMID 5446326.
120 Kehoe, P. et al., *'Is inhibition of the renin-angiotensin system a new treatment option for Alzheimer's disease?'*, *Lancet neurol.*, 6(4) 2007, 373–78, PMID 17362841.
121 BBC 4, June 2007, *'Why stroke ups Alzheimer's risk'* (http//news.bbc.co.uk/1/hi/health/6713163.stm).
122 Hawkes, N., *'Alzheimers linked to aluminium pollution in tap water'*, *The Times*, 20 April 2006 (http://www.timesonline.co.uk/tol/news/uk/health/article707311.ece).
123 Rondeau, V. et al., *'Relation between drinking water and Alzheimer's disease: an 8-year follow-up study'*, *Am.j.epidemiol.* 169/4) 1008, 489–96, PMID 19064650.
124 Yumoto, S. et al., *'Demonstration of aluminium in amyloid fibers in the cores of senile plaques in the brains of patients with Alzheimer's disease'*, *J. of inorganic biochemistry*, 103 (11) 2009, 1579–84, PMID 19744735.
125 Ferreira, P. C. et al., *'Aluminium as a risk factor for Alzheimer's disease'*, *Rev. Lat. Am. Enfermagem*, 16 (1) 2008, 151–157, PMID 18392545.
126 Bundesinstitut für Risikobewertung, *'Aluminium-haltige Antitranspirantien tragen zur Aufnahme von Aluminium bei'*, 10 March 2010 (http://www.

bfr.bund.de/cm/343/aluminiumhaltige-antitranspirantien-tragen-zur-aufnahme-von-aluminium-bei, PDF,15 pages).

127 Linn, T.T. et al., *"The 'preclinical phase' of probable Alzheimer's disease: a 13-year prospective study of the Framingham cohort"*, Arch.neuro.52 (5) 1995, 485–90, PMID 7733843.

128 Saxton, Y. et al., *'Preclinical Alzheimer's disease: neuropsychological test performance 1.5 to 8 year prior onset'*, Neurology 63 (12) 2004, 2341–2347, PMID 15623697.

129 Twamley, E.W. et al., *'Neuropsychological and neuroimaging changes in preclinical Alzheimer's disease'*, J.int.neuropsychol soc., 12 (5) 2006, 707–735, PMID 16961952.

130 Sperling, R.A. et al., *'Toward defining the preclinical stages of Alzheimer's disease: recommendations from the National Institute on Aging – Alzheimer's Association workgroup on diagnostic guidelines for Alzheimer's disease'*, Alzheimer's & Dementia, vol. 7 (3) May 2011, 280–92, PMID 21514248.

131 Albert, M.S. et al., *'The diagnosis of mild cognitive impairment due to Alzheimer's disease: recommendations from the National Institute on Aging – Alzheimer's Association workgroups on diagnostic guidelines for Alzheimer's disease'*, J. Alzheimer's Ass., vol. 7 (3) 2011, 270–79, PMID 21514249.

132 Gertz, H.I. et al., *'Diagnose ohne Therapie. Frühdiagnostik der Alzheimer-Krankheit im Stadium der leichten kognitiven Beeinträchtigung'*, Der Nervenarzt, vol. 82 (9) 2011, PMID 21481640.

133 Barthel, J. et al., *'Cerebral amyloid-β PET with florbetaben (18F) in patients with Alzheimer's disease and healthy controls: a multicentre phase 2 diagnostic study'*, Lancet Neurol, vol. 10 (5) May 2011, 424–35, PMID 21481640.

134 Mucke, L., *'Alzheimer's disease'*, Nature 461, 2009, 895–7, PMID 19829367.

135 Förstl, H. et al., *'Clinical features of Alzheimer's disease'*, European Arch of Psychiatry and clinical neuroscience, vol. 249 (6) 1999, 288–90, PMID 10653284.

136 Frank, E.M. et al., *'Effect of Alzheimer's disease on communication function'*, J of the South Carolina Medical Association, 1975, vol. 90 (9) 1994, 417–23, PMID 7967534.

137 Becker, J.T. et al., *'The semantic memory deficit in Alzheimer's disease'*, Revista de Neurologia, vol. 35 (8) 2002, 777–83, PMID 12402233.

138 Hodges, J.R. et al.,*'Is semantic memory consistently impaired early in the course of Alzheimer's disease? Neuroanatomical and diagnsic implications'*, Neuropsychologia, vol. 33 (4) 1995, 441–59, PMID 7617154.

139 Benke, T., *'Two forms of apraxia in Alzheimer's disease'*, Cortex, a J. Devoted to the Study of the Nervous System and Behavior, vol. 29 (4) 1993, 715–25, PMID 8124945.

140 Förstl H. et al., *'Clinical features of Alzheimer's disease'*, Eur Arch Psychiatry a Clinical Neuroscience, vol. 249 (6) 1999, 288–90, PMID 10653284.

141 Carlesimo, G.A. et al.,*'Memory deficits in Alzheimer's patients: a comprehensive review'*, Neuropsychology rev., vol. 3(2) 1992, 119–69, PMID 1300219.

142 Kumru, L., *'Getting Lost in Alzheimer's'*, UNMC, downloaded 22 July 2007 (https://web.archive.org/web/20010510071335/http://www.unmc.edu/publicaffairs/discover/fall99stories/alzheimer).

143 (http://alzheimer-forschung.de/forschung/aktuelles.htm? Showid=3237), 'Zukunftsmusik? Impfung gegen das Vergessen', 6. Oct 2010, downloaded 5 Oct 2010.

144 Wirths, O. et al.,*'Identification of low molecular weight pyroglutamate A(beta)oligomers in Alzheimer disease: a novel tool for therapy and diagnosis'*, J of Biological Chemistry, vol. 285 (53), 2010, 41517–41524, PMID 20971852.

145 Weller, S. et al., *'Therapie gegen Alzheimer: Göttinger Forscher entwickeln neuen Ansatz für passive Immunisierung'*, Universitätsmedizin Göttingen, Georg August Universität, press release of 5 Nov. 2010, Informationsdienst Wissenschaft (idw-online.de), downloaded 6 Nov 2010.

146 Studeny, J., *'Drug quickly reverses Alzheimer's symptoms in mice'*, Case Western Univerity, 9 Feb 2002/12 (http://www.eurokalert.org/pub_releases/2012-02/cwru-dqr020512.php).

147 Meldung Nuerosciencenews.com, 10 Feb 2012: *'Drug quickly Reverses Alzheimer's Symptoms in Mice'*, (http://neurosciencenews.com/alzheimers-disease-canccer-drug-bexarotene/).

148 Frater, H., *'Krebsmedikament macht Alzheimer-Symptome rückgängig: Wirkstoff Bexaroten beseitigt Gedächtnisstörungen und Eiweiss-Plaques

bei Mäusen', in g.o.de. 10 Feb 2012, downloaded 27 Dec 2014 (http://www.g.o.de/wissen-aktuell-14430-2012-02-10.html).
149 Francis, P. W. et al., 'The cholinergic effect hypothesis of Alzheimer's disease: a review of progress', J Neurol Neurosurg Psychiatry 1999 (http://jnnp.bmj.com/content/66/2/137.full*ref-8).
150 Lempert, T. et al., 'Treatment of Alzheimer's disease according to the S3 guidelines on dementia. Cholin esterase inhibitors for all and forever?', Der Nervenarzt, vol. 82 (1) Jan 2011, 90–91, PMID 21274696.
151 Breitner, J. C. et al., 'Delayed onset of Alzheimer's disease with nonsteroidal anti-inflammatory and histamine H2 blocking drugs',. Neurobiology of Aging, vol. 16 (4) 523–30, July 1995, PMID 8544901.
152 Wyss-Coray, T. et al., 'Ibuprofen, inflammation and Alzheimer's disease', Nature medicine, vol. 6 (9), Sept 2000, 973–74, PMID 10973311.
153 Dokmeci, D., 'Ibuprofen and Alzheimer's disease', Folia medica, vol. 46 (2), 2004, 5–10, PMID 15506544.
154 Morihara, T. et al., 'Ibuprofen suppresses interleukin-I-beta induction of pro-amyloidogenic alpha 1-antichymotrypsin to ameliorate beta-amyloid (Abeta) pathology in Alzheimer's models', Neuropsychopharmacology: official publication of the American college of neuropsychopharmacology, vol. 30 (6) June 2005, 1111–1120, PMID 15688088.
155 McKee, A.C. et al., 'Ibuprofen reduces Abeta, hyperphosphorylated tau and memory deficits in Alzheimer mice', Brain research, vol. 1207, May 2008, 225–236, PMID 18374096.
156 Sastre, M. et al., 'Nonsteroidal anti-inflammatory drugs repress beta-secretase gene promoter activity by the activation of PPARgamma', Proceedings of the National Academy of Sciences of the United States of America, vol. 103 (2) Jan 2006, 443–8, PMID 16407166.
157 Tabet, N. et al., 'Ibuprofen for Alzheimer's disease', Cochrane database of systematic reviews, no. 2 2003, CD004031, doi:10.100214651858. CD004031, PMID 12804498.
158 De Strooper, D. et al., 'An antiinflammatory drug prospect', Nature, vol. 414(6860) Nov 2001, 159–60, PMID 11700538.
159 Larbig, G., 'Studien zur Identifizierung & Optimierung potentieller Wirkstoffe für die Behandlung von Morbus Alzheimer', dissertation, Darmstadt Tech Univ, 2007 (http./elib.tu-darmstadt.de/diss/000827).
160 Müller, T., 'Neue Wege gegen das Amyloid im Hirn', Deutsche Ärztezeitung, 7 Dec 2007 (http://www.aerztezeitung.de/medizin/krankheiten/demenz/?sid=473993).
161 Krohn, M. et al., 'Cerebral Amyloid-β proteostasis is regulated by the membrane transport protein ABCC 1 in mice', J of clinical investigation, vol. 121 (10) Oct 2011, 3924–31.
162 Chane, M. et al., 'Memantine for dementia', The Cochrane database of systematic reviews, no. 2, 2006, CD003154, PMID 16625572.
163 Krishnan, S. et al., 'Cannabinoids for the treatment of dementia', The Cocchraine database of systemic reviews, no. 2, 2009, CD007204. pub2), PMID 19370677.
164 Craft, S. et al., 'Intranasal insulin therapy for Alzheimer disease and amnestic mild cognitive impairment: a pilot clinical al.', Arch neurology, vol. 69 (1) Jan 2012, 29–39.
165 Birks, J. et al., 'Ginkgo biloba for cognitive impairment and dementia', Cochrane Database Syst Rev, CD003120, PMID 12519586.
166 Birks, J. et al., 'Ginkgo biloba for cognitive impairment and dementia', Cocchrane Database Syst Rev, 2, 2007, CD003120, PMID 17443523.
167 Dysken, M. W. et al., 'Affect of vitamin E and memantine on functional decline in Alzheimer disease: the TEAM-AD V A cooperative randomized trial', JAMA, vol. 311 (1), Jan 2014, 33–44, PMID 4109898.
168 Sano, M. et al.,'A controlled trial of selegiline, alpha-tocopherol, or both as treatment for Alzheimer's disease: the Alzheimer's disease Cooperative Study', New Engl J of Medecine, vol. 335 (17), April 1997, 1216–1222, PMID 9110909.
169 Peterson, R. C. et al., 'Vitamin E Donepezil for the treatment of mild cognitive impairment', New Engl J of Medicine, vol. 352 (23), June 2005, 2379–2388.
170 Kang, J. H. et al.,'A randomized trial of vitamin E supplementation and cognitive function in women', Archives of internal medicine, vol. 166(22), 2006 Dec 11–25, 2462–68.
171 Kang, J. H. et al., 'Vitamin E, vitamin C beta caro-

tene, and cognitive function among women with or at risk of cardiovascular disease', Circulation, vol. 119(21), June 2009, 2772–80, PMID 19451353.

172 Miller, E. R. et al., 'Meta-analysis: high-dosage vitamin E supplementation may increase all-cause mortality', Ann of internal medicine, vol. 142 (1), Jan 2005, 37–46, PMID 15537682.

173 Guo, J. P. et al., 'Simple in vitro assays to identify amyloid-beta aggregation blockers for Alzheimer's disease therapy', J. Alzheimers Dis., 19 (4) 2010, 1359–70, PMID 20061605.

174 Abbas, S. et al., 'Epigallocatechin gallate inhibits beta amyloid oligomerization in Caenorhabditis elegans and effects the daf-2/insulin-like signaling pathway', J Alzheimers Dis., 17 (11) 2010, 902–9, PMID 20382008.

175 Ehrnhoefer, D. E. et al., 'DGCG redirects amyloidogenic polypeptides into unstructured, off-pathway oligomers', Nat Struct Mol Biol., 15 (5) June 2008, 558–566, PMID 18511942.

176 Bieschke, J. et al., 'EGSG remodels mature α-synuclein and amyloid-β-fibrils and reduces cellular toxicity', Proc Natl Acad Sci USA, 107 (17) April 2010, PMID 20385841.

177 Meng, F. et al., 'The Flavanol(-) epigallocatechin 3-gallate inhibits amyloid formation by islet amyloid polypeptide , disaggregates amyloid fibrils, and protects cultural cells against IAPP-induced toxicity', Biochemistry, 49 (37), Sept 2010, PMID 20707388.

178 Rezai-Zadeh, K. et al., 'Green tea epigallocatechin-3-gallate (EGCG) reduces beta-amyloid mediated cognitive impairment and modulates tau pathology in Alzheimer transgenic mice', Brain Res, 12(1214), June 2008, 177–86, PMID 18457818.

179 Charité Berlin, 'Wie greift EGCG in den Mechanismus der Amyloidbildung ein?', http://www.hunstein-egcg.de/Bieschke-de.html).

180 Greeke, G. et al., 'Black tea theaflavins inhibit formation of toxic amyloid-β-and α-synuclein fibrils', Biochemistry, Nov 2011, PMID 22054421.

181 Gary, W. et al., 'What we need to know about age related memory loss', Brit. Med. J., 22 June 2002 (http://bmjjournals.com/cgi/content(full/324/7352/1502), downloaded 5 Nov 2006.

182 Scalco, M. Z. et al., 'Prevention of Alzheimer's disease: encouraging evidence', Canadian family physician, vol. 52, Feb 2006, 300–307, PMID 16529393.

183 Scalco, M. Z. et al., 'Prevention of Alzheimer's disease: encouraging evidence', Canadian family physician, vol. 52, Feb 2006, 200–207, PMID 16529393.

184 Watzel, B. and Leitzmann, C., Bioaktive 'Substanzen in Lebensmitteln', Hippokrates-Verlag, Stuttgart, ISBN 3 7773-1115-4, 1995.

185 Becher, G. R. et al., 'Analysis of micronutrients in foods', in Moon, T. E. and Micozzi, M. S. (eds), 'Nutrition and cancer prevention: investigating the roles of micronutrients', Decker, New York, 1988, 103–58.

186 Hertog, M. G. et al., 'Optimization of a quantitative HPLC-determination of potentially anticarcinogenic flavonoids in vegetables and fruits', J.Agric Food chem., 40 (1992), 1591–6.

187 Billings et al., 'Inhibition of radiation-induced transformation of CH3/10T1/2-cells by chymotrypsin-inhibitor 1 from potatoes', Carcinogenesis 8, 1987, 809–12.

188 Steinmetz, K. A. et al., 'Vegetables, fruit and cancer I and II', Epidemiology, Cancer Causes Control, 2 (1991a), 325–57.

Index

α-carotene	65	Alzheimer's disease	7, 8, 12, 20, 29, 30, 32, 34, 44, 45, 46, 57
β-amyloid	29, 30, 32, 45, 52, 57, 58, 59	– causes	57
β-carotene	65	– change of character in	61
		– deterioration, physical, in	62
Ability to focus, reduced	36	– determining the diagnosis	60
Ability to learn	35, 61	– dietary treatment	65
Ability to speak	61	– differential diagnosis	60
Abscesses of the tooth roots, effect for the brain	19	– genetics	58
Acetylcholine	15, 37, 40	– life expectancy in	62
Acetylcholinesterase inhibitors	62	– occurrence (prevalence), frequency, age	57
Acid-base balance in the brain	16	– occurrences in the brain	59
Acrodynia (Feer's disease)	34	– officially recognised risks of	64
ACTH (adrenocorticotropic hormone)	13	– preclinical stage	60
ADAM 10, ADAM 17	59	– prophylaxis of	62
Adenohypophysis (anterior lobe of the hypophysis)	13	– stage of mild cognitive impairment (MCI)	60
Adenosine	41	– stages of	61
Adenosine triphosphate (ATP)	59	– treatment, medication	62
ADH (antidiuretic hormone, vasopressin)	14, 16	Amalgam fillings and neurotoxicity	33
		Amphetamines	39
ADHS (Attention Deficit Hyperactivity Syndrome)	41	Amyloid precursor protein (APP)	59
		Amyotrophic lateral sclerosis (ALS)	32, 46
Adrenaline	15, 40, 44	Anterior lobe of the hypophysis (adenohypophysis)	13
Afterbrain (myelencephalon)	11	Anthocyanin	66
Agnosia (inability to recognise objects)	49	Antibodies, monoclonal	62
		Antidiuretic hormone	14
AIDS and dementia	50	Antigen-presenting cells in the brain	16
Alcohol syndrome, foetal	41	Antioxidative potential	65
Alcohol, toxicity	41	Anxiety	36, 51, 54
Allergic diseases of the IV-type	34	Aphasia (inability to speak)	49, 52, 61
Allergies	34	Apoptosis (cell death)	32, 34, 37, 60
Allicin	67	APP-1	59
Alpha secretase	59	Appetite	34
Alpha-synuclein	9, 30, 64	Apraxia (inability to perform movements correctly)	49, 61
Aluminium and Alzheimer's disease	58	Aquaporins	18
Alzheimer Alois	7	Arteriosclerosis	7, 44
Alzheimer's dementia	9, 35		

Art therapy	54	Carvone	67
AS-amyloidosis	26	Catalase	31
Astrocytes	16, 17, 18, 29	Cationic transport through	
Ataxia	48	blood-brain barrier	18
Atrophy of the brain in		Caudate nucleus	11
Alzheimer's disease	60	Cell receptor LINGO1	24
Autisms	12, 34	Cell respiration	59
Autoimmune	34	Cerebellum	11
Autoimmune inflammations	44	Cerebral cortex (archipallium)	12
Autoimmune processes	7, 29, 30, 68	Cerebral immune system	66
Avolition	37	Cerebrum (cortex)	10
Axon	10, 15, 29	Change of character in dementia	51, 61
		Change of personality in dementia	36
Background stress, toxic	36	Chaos principle (Clausius)	28, 65
Basal ganglia	11	Chaperones	32
Basic regulation system (Pischinger)	29	Chemical transmitters	15
Batteries, toxicity	37	Chemokine CXCL12	24
Benzo[a]pyrene	41	Chewing, a risk factor for dementia	51
Benzodiazepines (sleeping pills		Chloride radical (Cl*)	32
of the Valium group)	12, 16	Chlorinated hydrocarbons, toxicity	19
Beta amyloid	29, 30, 57, 58	Chlorine and neurodegenerative	
– creation of	59	diseases	35
Beta-endorphin	40	Chlorophyll α molecules	27
Bexarotene	62	Choking seizures	36
Black core (nucleus niger)	11	Cholesterol	15, 22, 58
Black tea, effect of theaflavin	63	Chorea Huntington	50
Blood-brain barrier	17, 29	Chorea minor	12
Blood pressure	18	Choreatic disorder	12
Blood pressure in the brain	18	Chrome	37
Brain plasticity	14	Cleaning agents, toxicity	35
Brain tumour and dementia	61	Cocaine	40
Breast milk, flame retardants	37	Coherence	27
Breathing, acute problems	36	Coherence principle of Prigogine	28
Bridge	11	Combined effect of harmful	
Bromide radical (Br*)	32	neurotoxic substances	42
Bullying	46	Complex IV of the respiration chain,	
Butyrophenone, toxicity	37	block of the	59
		Connexin (CX32)	22
CADASIL disease	49	Conscious mind	11
Cadmium	37	Controlling emotions	10
Calcium	15, 33	Cooking, loss of effect by	65, 66
Calories, importance	27	Copper, neurotoxicity	33
Canal proteins in the		Corpora amygdalae	12
blood-brain barrier	18	Corpus callosum	10
Cancer, development of cancer cells	31	Corpus mamillare	12
Cancer risk, coffee	42	Corpus striatum (striped core)	11
Cannabis	39, 63	Corticothalamic system	11
Cardiac centre	11	Cortisol	13, 42
Carotenoids	65	Coughing reflex	11

Cramps and organic tin compounds	34	Dietary treatment of neurodegenerative diseases	65
Creutzfeldt-Jakob's disease	50	Diethylperazine	63
Cyclothymia (manic-depressive disorder)	61	Diphenyl ether, polybromated (PBDE)	37
Cytochrome C	32	Disease definition (Bircher-Benner)	28
Cytochrome P 450-oxidase	31	Disinfectant	35
Cytokines	17, 19, 24, 34, 42	Disinhibition in dementia	51
		Dissipative system (Prigogine)	28
Damage to the memory	36	Distrust in dementia	51
Decisions	10	Disturbances of the lipid metabolism, congenital forms and dementia	50
Delirium in dementia	52	DNA peroxidation	31
Delusions in dementia	51	Dopamine	38, 40
Dementia	49	Down's syndrome (trisomy 21) and Alzheimer's dementia	58
– as a consequence of other general diseases	50	Driving cars and dementia	55, 56
– degenerative forms of dementia	49	Drugs, legal and prohibited	39
– diagnosis	49, 52	Dysexecutive syndrome	49
– early recognition of the onset of dementia	52, 60		
– forms of dementia	49	E4 allele of apolipoprotein E (Apo E)	58
– forms of genetically inherited vascular dementia	49	Effect of alcohol consumption on the blood-brain barrier	19
– frequency (prevalence) and age at onset	50	Effect of electromagnetic radiation on the human brain	20
– informing the patient	53	Effect of smoking on the blood-brain barrier	20
– legal issues	55	Electroencephalogram and spectra of the sunlight	21
– risk factors, accepted, for dementia	50	Electromagnetic radiation, effect on the brain	30, 44, 46
– risk reduction, means for	55	Ellagic acid	66
– stage of mild cognitive impairment (MCI)	52	Emaciation in dementia (marasmus)	51
– symptoms of dementia	51	Encephalopathy	48
– vascular dementia	49	Encephalopathy, toxic	35
Demyelinating diseases	23	Energy, chaotic, orderly	27
Dendrites	14	Environmental stress and neurogenerative diseases	33
Deoxyribonucleic acid DNA, hereditary material	27	Epigallocatechin gallate (EGCG, green tea)	63
Depression	12, 16, 36, 50, 51, 52, 54, 61	Epiphysis	14
		Erectile problems	26
Deprivation and pseudodementia	52, 61	Euphoria (unnaturally high mood) in dementia	51
Detoxification enzymes	31	Executive cortex	10
Development of consciousness	11	Exhaustion (cronic fatigue Syndrome)	42
Diabetes mellitus	44, 51, 58	Exposure to the sun	44, 67
Diabetic neuropathy	32	Eyes, irritation	36
Dialysis treatment, long-standing effect on the brain	25		
Dichlorfluanid	37		

Factor EGF	24	Hair analysis	34
Faraday cage, ineffectiveness mobile phone signals	20	Hallucinations in dementia	51, 52
		Headache by toxic substances	42
Fatigue, chronic (chronic fatigue syndrome)	36	Headache caused by toxic substances	36
		Head trauma and Alzheimer's risk	58, 61
Fatty acids, polyunsaturated (PUFA)	18	Hearing damage through toxins	36
		Heart attack, risk, coffee	42
Feer's disease (acrodynia)	34	Heavy metals, toxic	30
Fibrils, twisted	29, 60	HERNS syndrome	49
Flame retardants	37	Heroin	40
Flavonoids	63, 65, 66	High blood pressure, hypertonia	42
Flaxseed oil	67	Hiking, effect	54
Fluid balance in the brain	16	Hippocampus	9, 10, 12, 35, 37, 52, 60, 61
Focused, targeted thinking and decision-making	10	Hives (urticaria)	34
Folding sheet structures	25	Homeostasis, regulation of the, in the brain	18
Folic acid, 5 methyltetrahydrofolic acid (5-MTHF)	44, 52, 67	Homocysteine	44, 51, 52
Food energy	27	Homunculus	10
Fornix	12	Hormone-producing glands	13
Free radicals	31, 65, 67	Hospitalism	61
Frontotemporal dementia (PICK's disease)	52	Huntington's disease	12, 32
		Hydrocarbons, volatile, organic	36
FSH (follicle stimulating hormone)	13	Hydrogen peroxide (H_2O_2)	31
		Hydroxyl radical (OH*)	31
GABA (γ-aminobutyric-acid)	16	Hyperactivity	34
Galactocerebroside	22	Hyperaesthesia (excessive pain sensitivity)	35
Galacto-sulfatide	22	Hyperpathia (oversensitivity)	35
Gene for APO-E	58	Hyperphosphorylation	60
GH (somatotropin or growth hormone)	14	Hypertension	58
Ginkgo biloba	63	Hypertension and risk of dementia	58
Glia	10, 15, 16, 33	Hypertonia	42
Glial cells	29	Hypochlorites (swimming pools)	35
Glial scars	16, 17	Hypothalamus	13
Globus pallidus (pale core)	11, 12	Hypothyreosis and dementia	50
GLUT-1 transporter	18		
Glutamate	15, 16, 32, 37	Ibuprofen and Alzheimer's disease	62
Glutathione	31, 44	Immune competence	29
Glutathione reductase	31	Immune defence of the brain	16
Glutathione-S-transferase	67	Immune system, enteral	68
Glycine	16	Immunological barrier to the brain	17
GPS localization system to find patients who have run away	54	Impaired sensation	34
		Impairment of memory	51, 60
Green tea	63	Impairment of short-term memory	51
Grey matter	10, 14	Inability to assess emotional situations	12
Gyri	10		
Gyrus cinguli	12	Incontinence as an early sign of the onset of dementia	51

Infant death, sudden and amalgam fillings	33
Infection hypothesis on Alzheimer's dementia	58
Infusion therapy, antioxidative	53
Insomnia	34
Insulin	63
Insulin resistance and Alzheimer's disease	58
Insurance matters in case of dementia	56
Interferon γ	17
Interleukin-1	17
Interleukin IL1-α	19, 35
Interleukin IL1-β	19
Interleukin IL-6	19, 35
Intestinal flora, importance with regards to dementia	68
Irritability	42
Irritation, chronic	36
Javelle water	35
Kinks	18
Lab control recommendations for the attending physician	68
Lack of appetite	34
Lack of movement and dementia	51
Language centre (Broca Wernicke's area)	10
LASER amplification of the UV light in the cells	20, 27, 65
LASER threshold	27
LDL cholesterol	18
L-dopa	52
Lead	37
Learning	14
Learning aptitude	41
Lecithin	22
Legal guardianship and dementia	55
Leukodystrophies	22
Lewy body dementia	32, 49, 52
LH (luteinising hormone)	13
Light, oversensitivity of the skin	36
Limbic system	12, 35
Limonene	67
LINGO1 receptors	24
Lipid peroxidation	31, 32, 37
Lipophilin	22
Liquor cerebrospinalis	17
Living will	55
Loss of coordination of movement (ataxia)	36
LSD (lysergic acid diethylamide)	39
Lupus erythematosus	50
Lutein	65
Lycopene	65
Lymphatic system	29
Lysergic acid diethylamide (LSD)	39
Macrophages	16
Magnesium	15
Maintenance of the homeostasis in the brain	16
MAK limits, too high	36
Manic-depressive psychosis (cyclothymia)	51, 61
Marasmus (emaciation), in dementia	51
Matrix (intracellular substance)	29
MCT-1 and MCT-2 transport systems	18
Medicines, neurotoxic effects	37, 42
Medulla oblongata	11, 40
Melatonin	14
Memory problems	12
Memory, strengthening	11
Memory training	54
Meningea arachnoidea (spider-web-like cerebral membrane)	17
Meningitis, risk through smoking	20
Mental confusion	34
Mental illness (psychoses)	52, 61
Mental performance, reduced	42
Menus	72
Mercury and Alzheimer disease	33
Mercury and -amyloid deposit	33
Mercury and neurodegenerative diseases	33
Mesencephalon (midbrain)	11
Metabolic syndrome and dementia	51, 58
Methionine, S-Adenosyl methionine	44
Methylmercury, neurotoxicity	34
Microangiopathic lesions	49
Microglia	17, 29, 66
Microglial cells	16
Micro-vascular changes	49
Mid brain (Mesencephalon)	11
Migraines	42
Miscolonisation, enteral	68

119

Mitochondria	31, 59	Neurovascular unit	19
Mobile phones and the brain	20	Niacin deficit	50
Morphine	40	Nicastrin	59
Morphogenetic fields	20	Nickel	37
Motion control	12	Nicotine	40
Motoneuron, 1 and 2	13	Nicotine during pregnancy	41
Motoric end plate		Nitric oxide	19
(transfer point nerve muscle)	15	Nitric oxide radical (NO*)	32
Motoric pathways	12	Nitrosative stress	32, 34
Mould	33	Nitroxygen (NO*)	31
Movement training in dementia	54	NMDA receptor antagonists	63
MSH (melanocyte-stimulating		NMDA receptor	
hormone)	14	(N-methyl-D-aspartate receptor)	32, 37
Multi-infarct syndrome	49	Nodes of Ranvier	15
Multiple chemical sensitivity, MCS	35	Non-steroidal antirheumatics	
Multiple sclerosis	8, 9, 17, 19, 20, 23, 24, 29, 30, 32, 46, 50	(NSAR)	62
		Noradrenaline	15, 40, 44
Multiple system atrophy (MSA)	7, 9, 52	NO-synthase	32
Muscarinic receptors	37	Notch-1 receptors	24
Muscle weakness	35	Nuclei pontis	11
Music therapy	54	Nucleus niger (black core)	11
Mutism (refusal to speak)	52, 61	Nucleus subthalamicus	12
Myelencephalon (afterbrain)	11	Nursing aids for patients	
Myelin	16	with dementia	55
Myelin basic protein (MBP)	22		
Myelin marrow sheaths	22	Obesity and dementia	38
Myelin oligodendrocyte glycoprotein		Oestrogens	13
(MOG)	22	Olfactory bulb	10
Myelin protein, basic (MBP)	22	Oligodendrocytes	22
Myelin sheaths	14, 34, 37	Oligodendroglia	16, 29
Myosin light-chain enzyme (MLCK)	20	Omega-3-fatty acids	67
Myosin light-chain kinase (MLCK)	19	Omega-6-fatty acids	67
		Opiates	40
		Organic phosphorus pesticides	36
NADH (nicotinamide adenine		Oxidative stress	20, 31, 32, 34, 44, 51, 59, 63, 65
dinucleotide hydrogen)	44		
Nails, growth impairment	36		
Narcolepsy (inadvertent sleeping		Oxytocin	14, 16
during the day)	12		
Nausea, constant	36	Pale core (globus pallidus)	11
Nerve cell (neuron)	14, 15	Palsy, progressive, supranuclear	52
Nervous system is overstimulated	15	Panarteritis nodosa	50
Neurites	10	Paralysis	36
Neurodegenerative diseases	47	Paraplegia	16
Neurodermitis and mercury	34	Parkinson's disease	9, 12, 15, 32, 34, 38, 46, 51, 52
Neuroleptics	12		
Neuron (nerve cells)	10		
Neuropathy, peripheral	36	Patients with dementia running away	54
Neurotransmitters	15	PEN-1, PEN-2	59

Pentachlorophenol (PCP)	37	Protease inhibitors	66
Pericytes	18	Protein hyperphosphorylation	
Peripheral neuropathy	26	of the TAU-protein	33
Peroxide dismutase	31	Protein peroxidation	31
Peroxynitrite	32	Protein zero (P0, MPZ)	22
Pesticides and neurodegenerative		Proteolipid protein (PLP/DM20)	22
diseases	44	PSEN 1 (presenilin 1),	
PET (positron emission tomography)	52, 61	PSEN 2 (presenilin 2)	58
P-glycoprotein system	19	Psychoses (mental illness)	61
PgP receptor	19	Putrefaction toxins	68
Phagocytosis (absorption by cells)	25	Pyrethroid, semi-synchronistic	37
Phase II enzymes of detoxing		Pyroglutamate Abeta	62
in the intestinal mucosa	66		
Phenoloxidase	66	Quercetin	66
Phenothiazine	37	Quinones	66
Phobias	12		
Phosphatidylethanolamine	22	Radicals, free	31, 60
Phosphorylation	8	Ratio of omega-3 to omega-6	67
Photon	20	Rauwolfia, toxicity	38
Phytochemicals	65	Raw food therapy, practical application	72
Pick's disease	50, 52	Rear strands in the rear spinal cord	13
Pink disease	34	Recipes	76
Pituicytes	16	Reduction of risk, means for,	
Plexus choroideus		in dementia	55
(secretes the brain fluid)	17	Remyelination	24
Pollutants and neurogenerative		Renal insufficiency and dementia	72
diseases	33	Reserpine	38
Polyneuropathy	35	Resilience, reduced mental and	
Polyneuropathy, peripheral	34	emotional	35
Polyphenols	66	Respiratory centre	11
Polyunsaturated fatty acids	15	Respiratory chain, chemical,	
Pons	11	in the mitochondria	31
Poor nutrition and neurodegeneration	46	Resting potential	15
Posterior horn of the spinal cord	13	Restlessness	42, 54
Posterior pituitary (neurohypophysis)	14	Rheumatic inflammations	44
Post-traumatic stress disorders	12	Rheumatism-like muscle pain	
Potassium	15, 16, 17, 33	(myalgia)	36
Potential for action	15	R.O.S. (reactive oxygen species)	31, 32, 59
prefrontal cortex	40, 60	Rutin	66
Pre-frontal cortex	10		
Pregnancy and alcohol	41	Salinon poisoning (tin)	35
Pregnancy and smoking	41	Scalar waves (Tesla)	20
Presenilin 1 and 2	58, 59	Schizophrenia	12
Prigogine's coherence principle	65	Schwann cells	15, 22
Primary effects	42	Secondary effects	42
PRL (prolactin)	13	Secondary plant substances	65
Problem-solving skills	10	Second law of thermodynamics	
Processing of emotions	12	(Clausius)	28, 65
Prostaglandins	19	Secretase α	59

Selenium	31	Table on the general effect of	
Senile amyloidosis	26	raw food therapy	70
Sensitive tracks	13	Taking decisions	37
Sensitivity	10	TAU proteins	30, 57, 58, 60
Sensitivity to touch	35	Temporal lobes	10
Sensory cortex	10	Terpene	67
Septum pellucidum	12	Textiles, finishing, sports textiles,	
Serotonin	16, 40	toxicity	34
Short-term memory impairment	37	Thalamic nucleus	11, 13
Sick-Building Syndrome	36	Thallium	37
Silver, neurotoxicity	33	Theaflavin (black tea)	63
Singing, effect	14, 54	Thyroid hormones T3 and T4	13
Sleeping disorder	36, 51	Tight junctions	17, 18, 19
Sleeping disorders at night	42	Tin, neurotoxicity	33, 34
Sleeping pills	12	Toll-like receptors	24
Sleeping-waking rhythm	11	Tractus cerebrospinalis (nerve cords	
Sleep-wakefulness rhythm,		from the cortex to the spinal cord)	11
regulation of	46, 51	Tractus corticospinalis	
Smoking, toxicity	40, 51	(nerve pathways of the cortex	
Sneezing reflex	11	for motion control)	12
Sodium	15, 33	Transferrin, transport to the brain	18
Solvents, organic (VOC)	19	Transmembrane protein, type 1	59
SORL1 gene, mutation of the	58	Transport system through the	
Spaces of the brain	17	blood-brain barrier	18
Spatial memory	14	Transverse waves (Hertz)	20
Speech competence, promotion of	54	Trembling (tremor)	12, 52
STH	14	Tremor (trembling)	36, 52
Storage, loss of effect by	66	Tributyltin	34
Strategic legions	49	Trisomy 21 (Down's syndrome)	
Stress hormone axis, activation	42	and dementia	58
Striped core	11	TSH (thyroxine releasing hormone)	13
Stroke, risk, coffee	42	Tumour necrosis factor TNF	35
Substantia nigra (black matter)	12	TV, effect in dementia	55
Suicidal tendencies	37		
Sulci	10	Ubiquinone (of coenzyme Q10)	31
Sulphide	67	Ultraviolet light; UVB radiation	44
Sunlight	20, 27, 44	Underactivity of the thyroid gland	
Superoxide anion radical (O_2-)	31	and dementia	50
Swallowing reflex	11	Unmoral behaviour	37
Swimming pools, toxicity of the		Urge control	10, 36
treatment	35	UV light, storage of UV light	27
Synapses (connections between		UV light, UVA radiation	31
nerve cells)	15		
Syphilis	52	Vascular dementia (VAD)	7, 9, 44, 49, 61
Systematic overview of		Vasopressin	14
neurodegenerative diseases	47	Vegetable food, energy content	27
		Vegetable oils, polyunsaturated	
Table on the effects of foods on		(PUFA)	67
neurodegenerative diseases	69	Vegetables	88

Vertigo	36	White matter	10
Vesicular transport across the blood-brain barrier	18	White substance	22
		Wilson, Morbus	50
Vision problems through toxins	36	WLAN, effect on the brain	20
Visual cortex	10, 37	Wnt receptor	24
Vitamin A	31, 44, 67	Wood-protection agents, toxicity	36, 37
Vitamin antioxidative	31	Working memory, reduced	35, 36
Vitamin B1	41	Writing in the onset of dementia	61
Vitamin B6	44		
Vitamin B12	41, 44, 50, 52, 67	Xanthines	65
Vitamin C	31, 44, 66, 67	Zeaxanthin	65
Vitamin D	44, 45, 67	Zinc	44
Vitamin E	31, 67		
Vitamin K	44		
Vitamins antioxidative	44		

CENTRE FOR SCIENTIFIC NATURAL MEDICINE

SCIENTIFIC NATURAL MEDICINE
BIRCHER-BENNER
B R A U N W A L D

People come to the Bircher-Benner Medical Centre from a large number of countries in search of healing.

Here, you will be valued as a unique person, listened to and understood. Here, humanity and dignity are important and the medicine is a noble undertaking.

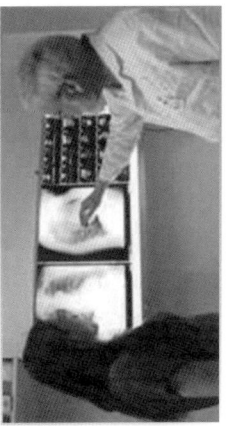

The search for the true causes of diseases is central to our work, as is the inclusion of your self-curative powers in the process of healing.

Centre for scientific natural medicine

Our fresh-vegetable diet will bring about a rapid change in your metabolism; natural regulative therapies take precedence where possible.

The atmosphere and the living tradition of the Bircher-Benner Centre, where novelty and modernity are combined with decades of experience, contribute to your healing.

The doctors and therapists will treat you personally and have all the facilities of a modern clinic at hand when needed.

The supplementation of traditional medicine by the regulative diagnosis and therapy of natural healing often permits a cure where the usual therapies have failed.

In the Medical Centre, you can relax and recover, and will experience the deep regeneration of your healing powers.

CENTRE BIRCHER-BENNER
CH-8784 Braunwald

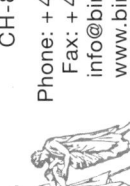

Phone: + 41 (0)21 801 60 04
Fax: + 41 (0)55 643 16 93
info@bircher-benner.com
www.bircher-benner.com

Indications: any internal diseases, migraine, tinnitus, neuralgia and other pain conditions, fibromyalgia, arthritis and arthrosis, collagenoses, liver, gallbladder and gastrointestinal diseases, metabolic diseases and diabetes, cardiovascular diseases, kidney and prostate diseases, women's diseases, allergies, skin diseases, convalescence, fatigue, depression and anxiety, menopausal, hormonal and weight problems.